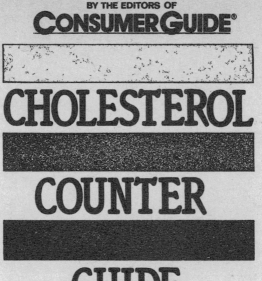

BY THE EDITORS OF
CONSUMER GUIDE®

CHOLESTEROL

COUNTER

GUIDE

Notice:
Neither the Editors of CONSUMER GUIDE® and Publications International, Ltd. nor the publisher take responsibility for any possible consequences from the use of the material in this publication. The publisher advises the reader to check with a physician before beginning any dietary program or therapy. This publication does not take the place of your physician's recommendations for diet modification. Every effort has been made to assure that the information in this publication is accurate and current at the time of printing.

Contents

Introduction

Why Worry About What You Eat?

Your diet affects more than your waistline. Your food choices and eating habits can greatly affect the health of your heart. Unfortunately, the damage that a poor diet does to your heart may not be as obvious as what it does to your figure—until it's too late.

The amount of cholesterol and fat in your diet can play a major role in the development of coronary heart disease, in which the arteries that supply the heart with blood become so narrowed with fatty deposits and blood clots that blood flow to the heart is restricted. Coronary heart disease is often called a "silent killer" because the deposits that clog the arteries develop gradually over the course of many years, often without giving you any warning. Sometimes, the first symptom of coronary heart disease is chest pain, known as "angina." Unfortunately, for some people, the first symptom is a fatal heart attack. A heart attack occurs when the blood flow to a portion of the heart is completely blocked and part of the heart muscle dies. If enough of the heart muscle is damaged, the victim dies. Heart attacks strike 1.5 million Americans each year and kill more than half of them.

Coronary heart disease is not limited to the elderly. Indeed, nearly half of all heart attacks occur in persons under the age of 65. What's more, the fatty deposits that may eventually block the artery can begin to develop as early as the childhood years. Fortunately, coronary heart disease is not an inevitable part of growing older. You can take steps now to help protect your heart and prevent the possibility of becoming a heart attack statistic.

While some of the factors that increase your risk of coronary heart disease, such as being male or having a family history of heart disease, are beyond your control, there are three major risk factors that you can control. The three major controllable risk factors for coronary heart disease are smoking, high blood pressure, and a high level of cholesterol in the blood. If you smoke, you *can* stop. If you have high blood pressure, you *can* work with your doctor to get it under control. Likewise, if you have a high blood cholesterol level, you *can* make dietary changes that can help to bring it down to a desirable level. Decreasing the amounts of saturated fat and cholesterol in your diet are the most important of those changes. And this book can help you make them.

What Is Cholesterol?

Cholesterol is a white, odorless, fat-like substance that is a basic component of the human body. Each of the body's cells is protected by a covering made up partly of cholesterol. As an essential part of the body's chemistry, cholesterol is used to produce the steroid hormones required for normal development and functioning. These include the sex hormones, which give men and women the physical traits characteristic of their sexes; cortisol, which is involved in regulating blood sugar levels and defending the body against infection; and aldosterone, which is important for retaining salt and water in the body. The body can also use cholesterol to make vitamin D, the vitamin responsible for strong bones and teeth, when the skin is exposed to sunlight.

Cholesterol is also used to make bile, a greenish fluid that is produced by the liver and stored in the gallbladder. The body needs bile to digest foods that contain fat and to absorb cholesterol from food. The body also needs bile to absorb vitamins A, D, E, and K, called fat-soluble vitamins, from foods or supplements. Indeed, cholesterol is so vital to our health that our bodies can make all the cholesterol we need.

INTRODUCTION

While our bodies have the ability to produce all the cholesterol we need, we can also get cholesterol from food. Cholesterol is found in many foods, although you can't taste it or see it on your plate. All animals have the ability to produce cholesterol, so all foods from animal sources, like milk, eggs, cheese, butter, and meat, contain cholesterol. Plants, on the other hand, do not manufacture cholesterol, so plant foods, like cereals, grains, nuts, fruits, and vegetables (and vegetable oils), do not contain cholesterol.

"Blood Cholesterol"

Some cholesterol is always present in the blood because the blood helps to transport cholesterol through the body. Cholesterol, however, is one of a group of substances known as lipids (fats), which do not dissolve in or mix with water. Therefore, in order to move the cholesterol through the bloodstream, the body wraps the cholesterol in protein, forming a molecule called a lipoprotein. The protein keeps the cholesterol from coming into contact with the blood and allows the cholesterol to be transported through the body.

Two types of lipoproteins play a major role in moving cholesterol through the blood. Low-density lipoproteins or LDLs carry cholesterol to the body's cells, where it can be used in a variety of ways. In contrast, high-density lipoproteins or HDLs are thought to carry cholesterol from the cells back to the liver so it can be removed from the body in the bile.

When more of the cholesterol in your blood is being carried by HDLs, there is less danger of cholesterol accumulating in the body, since HDLs are responsible for taking excess cholesterol to the liver where it can be excreted. That's why HDLs are often referred to as "good" cholesterol. If, on the other hand, most of the cholesterol in your blood is being carried by LDLs, more cholesterol may accumulate in the body. This is where the danger to your heart lies. The LDLs, which are often referred to as "bad" cholesterol, may take some of that unused cholesterol and deposit it in the walls of your coronary arteries (the vessels that carry oxygen-rich blood to the cells in your heart). Over time, this accumulation of cholesterol can begin to block the flow of blood to the heart. When that blood flow is completely cut off, some of the heart's cells suffocate and die. This is called a heart attack.

What Causes High Blood Cholesterol?

The body has several mechanisms that help it to balance the cholesterol it obtains from food with the cholesterol it produces. When your diet provides a substantial amount of cholesterol, your body decreases its own production of cholesterol. The body can also get rid of some excess cholesterol by using it to make bile and by dissolving some cholesterol in the bile that leaves the body through the feces.

These mechanisms aren't foolproof, however. In a very small minority of people (perhaps less than one percent of all those who have high blood cholesterol), an inherited defect can cause blood cholesterol levels to rise. This defect interferes with special receptor cells, located mainly on the surface of the liver, that are responsible for pulling cholesterol out of LDL molecules. When these receptors don't function properly, LDL-cholesterol is stranded in the bloodstream. As mentioned previously, a high level of LDL-cholesterol in the blood plays a major role in clogging arteries.

For the vast majority of people whose blood cholesterol levels are too high, however, the major culprits are high intakes of dietary cholesterol, saturated fat, and total fat. High intakes of dietary cholesterol and saturated fats can interfere with the functioning of the LDL receptors, causing a buildup of LDL-cholesterol in the blood.

A high intake of total fat appears to play a more indirect role. Since fat has more than twice the calories of carbohydrate and protein, a high-fat diet can provide more calories than the body requires. The unwanted calories are then stored in the body as fat. Over time, this can lead to overweight and obesity. Overweight, especially when it leads to obesity, appears to increase blood cholesterol levels. A high-fat diet is also likely to be high in saturated fats, which can increase blood cholesterol.

Is Your Blood Cholesterol Too High?

The level of cholesterol in your blood is expressed in "milligrams per deciliter (mg/dl)," which indicates the weight of the cholesterol found in one deciliter of blood. Research has shown that your risk of heart disease increases as your blood cholesterol level increases, especially as it rises past 200 mg/dl. In the United States, people who have a blood cholesterol level above 240 mg/dl appear to have more than twice the risk of developing coronary heart disease as do people whose blood cholesterol is below 200 mg/dl.

To help you and your physician determine if your blood cholesterol level puts you at high risk for coronary heart disease, the National Cholesterol Education Program (NCEP) recently developed recommendations for classifying cholesterol levels and determining treatment. The NCEP is a national partnership effort, coordinated by the federal government, involving 35 national medical, public health, and voluntary health organizations; one of it's major goals is to help educate the public about the importance of blood cholesterol. According to these recommendations, a total blood cholesterol level below 200 mg/dl is considered desirable for all adults over age 20. A total cholesterol level between 200 and 239 mg/dl is considered borderline-high and a total cholesterol level of 240 mg/dl or more is considered high. The recommendations specify that a total blood cholesterol measurement above 200 mg/dl must be confirmed by repeat testing.

If your blood cholesterol level is below 200 mg/dl, you should be given general dietary and risk-factor information and advised to have your cholesterol test repeated within five years. If your total cholesterol level is in the borderline-high range, you may need to be evaluated further, depending on whether you already have coronary heart disease or have two or more additional risk factors for the disease. Other risk factors include:

- Male gender
- Family history of premature (before age 55) coronary heart disease
- Cigarette smoking
- High blood pressure
- Low HDL-cholesterol level
- Diabetes
- Advanced hardening of the arteries
- Severe obesity (30 percent or more overweight).

If your total blood cholesterol is in the borderline-high range and you have no evidence of coronary heart disease and have fewer than two of these risk factors, you are advised to follow the *Step One* diet, which will be discussed in the next section. If your total blood cholesterol is in the borderline-high range and you have coronary heart disease or two or more risk factors for the disease, you are advised to have your lipoproteins measured. Likewise, if you have a high total blood cholesterol, you should have your lipoproteins evaluated. A lipoprotein analysis will reveal how your blood cholesterol is divided between LDL- and HDL-cholesterol.

If a lipoprotein analysis shows that your LDL level is below 130 mg/dl, you are advised to have your blood cholesterol tested again within five years. If your LDL level is 130 mg/dl or higher, however, you are advised to adopt the *Step One* diet.

Diets To Lower Blood Cholesterol
The *Step One* diet recommended by the NCEP to lower your blood cholesterol restricts your daily dietary

cholesterol intake to less than 300 milligrams. The diet also restricts your total fat intake to less than 30 percent of total calories and your saturated fat intake to less than ten percent of total calories. The remaining 20 percent of total calories from fat should be divided between mono-unsaturated and polyunsaturated fats.

If the *Step One* diet fails to lower your blood cholesterol to a desirable level, the *Step Two* diet is recommended. The *Step Two* diet restricts daily cholesterol intake to less than 200 mg daily and saturated fat intake to less than seven percent of total calories. The total fat allowance on this diet remains 30 percent since a diet that is much lower in fat would feel less filling and might therefore decrease patient compliance. In addition, a recent study has shown that lower total fat intakes are not necessary to adequately lower blood cholesterol.

Putting The Diets—And The Counter—To Work

To adopt the *Step One* diet, you need to be able to keep track of how much dietary cholesterol and fat you consume each day. This counter is designed to help you do just that. First, however, you need to look at what the dietary guidelines mean in terms of the foods you eat.

To limit your dietary cholesterol intake to less than 300 mg a day, you need to avoid or at least cut back on foods that are high in cholesterol. Remember that plants do not manufacture cholesterol, so foods that come from plants, like cereals, grains, fruits, and vegetables, do not contain cholesterol. Foods like eggs, dairy products, meats, poultry, and fish, which come from animal sources, contain varying amounts of cholesterol. The richest source of dietary cholesterol is the egg yolk, which contains about 250 mg of cholesterol. So experts recommend that you limit your egg yolk consumption each week to no more than two—and that's including yolks used in preparing foods.

To help you keep track of the cholesterol in foods and choose foods that are lowest in cholesterol, this counter shows you the cholesterol content of individual food items. The cholesterol (CHOL) content is listed in milligrams (mg). When you're planning your meals, you can simply add up the cholesterol values listed to find out if the foods you plan to eat will fit into your "daily cholesterol budget" of less than 300 mg (or less than 200 mg if you are on the *Step Two* diet). The counter can also help you compare similar foods so that you can opt for the item that is lower in cholesterol.

Both the *Step One* and the *Step Two* diets also restrict your total fat intake. Limiting your total fat intake will help you control your weight, which in turn can help you control your blood cholesterol. Limiting total fat intake can also help you to lower your saturated fat intake.

To help you limit your total fat intake to less than 30 percent of your total calories, this counter lists the total calories (CAL) and total fat (FAT) contained in individual foods. You can use these values to find out what percentage of a food's calories come from fat. The total fat for a food item is listed in grams (g). To figure out how many calories that translates into, you can multiply the number of grams by nine. You multiply by nine because every gram of fat—no matter where it comes from—provides your body with nine calories. So, for example, if a food lists it's total fat as eight grams and its total calories as 235, you would first multiply eight by nine. The resulting number, 72, tells you how many calories from fat (fat calories) the food provides. To determine what percentage of that food's total calories comes from fat, you simply divide the number of fat calories by the total number of calories and then multiply by 100. So you would divide 72 by 235, which equals .30, and then multiply by 100. Thus, 30 percent of that food's calories come from fat.

By choosing foods that get less than 30 percent of their calories from fat, you'll be able to limit your total fat intake. You don't have to eliminate all foods that get more than 30 percent of their total calories from fat. You should, however, try to at least cut back on them—serve them less often and in smaller portions. And when you do eat them, choose other foods that day that are low in fat. Keep in mind that you want your *overall* diet to provide less than 30 percent of your calories as fat.

The *Step One* diet further specifies what percentage of your fat calories should come from the three major types of fats: saturated, polyunsaturated, and monounsaturated. All living things have the ability to manufacture fat. Different species tend to manufacture different types of fats. In general, animals make a fat composed mainly of saturated fatty acids while plants tend to make fats composed mainly of polyunsaturated and monounsaturated fatty acids. The terms saturated and unsaturated refer to the number of hydrogen atoms found in the fatty acids that make up the fats. The degree of saturation determines whether the fat will be liquid or solid at room temperature, how useful it is in cooking, and how it affects your blood cholesterol levels.

Saturated fats are typically solid at room temperature. Butter, lard, and the marbling and visible fat in meats are saturated fats. Much of the fat in milk is also saturated and solid at room temperature, but the process of homogenization breaks the fat into fine particles and scatters it throughout the liquid portion of the milk. *Saturated fats tend to increase blood cholesterol because they interfere with the functioning of the receptors that pull LDL-cholesterol out of the bloodstream.*

Polyunsaturated fats are usually liquid at room temperature and are found mostly in the seeds of plants. The oils from safflowers, sunflowers, corn, soybeans, and cottonseed are polyunsaturated fats made up primarily of polyunsaturated fatty acids. *Polyunsaturated fats tend to lower blood cholesterol when they replace saturated fats in the diet. While polyunsaturated fats lower LDL levels, however, they also tend to lower HDL levels, although to a much lesser extent.*

Sometimes vegetable oils are chemically modified to change some of their polyunsaturated fatty acids to saturated ones. This process, called hydrogenation, is useful commercially because it improves the shelf life of the oils and allows the less expensive vegetable oils to acquire important baking properties that are normally found in the more costly animal fats. Hydrogenated or partially hydrogenated vegetable oils are more saturated than the original oils from which they're made. Margarine and vegetable shortening are examples of hydrogenated or partially hydrogenated vegetable oils.

Monounsaturated fats are also liquid at room temperature. Examples of fats rich in monounsaturated fatty acids are olive oil and rapeseed or canola oil. *Recent research appears to indicate that monounsaturated fats lower total blood cholesterol by lowering LDLs without lowering HDLs.*

Although most animal fats are usually saturated and most vegetable fats unsaturated, there are some noteworthy exceptions. Fish and chicken fats have fewer saturated fatty acids and more polyunsaturated fatty acids than do red meats such as beef, veal, lamb, and pork. The fat from fish is actually so rich in polyunsaturated fatty acids that it takes the form of an oil at room temperature just like fats usually found only in vegetables.

By the same token, a few vegetable fats are so rich in saturated fats that they are solid at room temperature. Palm oil, coconut oil, and palm kernel oil contain between 50 and 80 percent saturated fat. Coconut and palm oil are widely used in the commercial production of nondairy creamers, snacks such as popcorn and chips, baked goods, and candy. Cocoa butter, the fat found in some chocolates, is also rich in saturated fatty acids.

Foods rich in fat are usually those prepared by frying, basting, or marinating in butter, margarine, oil, or drippings from meat or poultry. Fat-rich foods can also be detected by their greasy texture. Sometimes, fat is visible, as in the whitish substance surrounding a steak or running through it. The fat in poultry is concentrated in the skin. Dairy products including whole milk, ice cream, and most cheeses are rich sources of saturated fats. Sometimes, however, it's hard to spot the fat in foods. For example, commercially prepared baked goods, like pies, cakes, and cookies, are common sources of "hidden fats." Although we may think of them only as sweets, they are often prepared with oils that are highly saturated.

Using this counter to choose foods that are low in cholesterol and total fat can also help you cut down on the amount of saturated fat you eat. Foods that are high in fat, especially if they come from animal sources, are often also high in saturated fats. Likewise, foods that are high in cholesterol also tend to be high in saturated fats. Remember that only animals produce cholesterol and that in general, animals tend to produce more saturated fatty acids than unsaturated ones. So if a particular product lists a high cholesterol content, chances are that much of the fat it contains is saturated. Exceptions to this include fish and poultry, which tend to produce higher amounts of polyunsaturated fatty acids. Shellfish, like lobster and shrimp, are rich in cholesterol but have a high content of polyunsaturated rather than saturated fat as well.

Foods that contain cholesterol and are also rich in saturated fat include beef, pork, veal, lamb, whole milk, cheese, cream, and ice cream. Sausages, luncheon meats, and frankfurters contain large amounts of total fat, saturated fat, and cholesterol. Commercially prepared baked goods, candy, and processed snack foods are frequently overlooked sources of considerable fat, saturated fat, and cholesterol. These "sweets" are often made with palm oil, coconut oil, or partially hydrogenated vegetable oils because these oils add flavor and are often cheaper than less saturated oils. Many of these products are also prepared with eggs. By eating fewer of these foods that are high in total fat and cholesterol, you can decrease the amount of saturated fat in your diet as well.

Here are some additional tips to help you choose and prepare foods that are low in saturated fat as well as cholesterol:

- Choose low-fat dairy products, such as skim milk, low-fat cottage cheese, nonfat yogurt, and ice milk, instead of whole milk, cream, hard cheese, sour cream, and ice cream.
- Choose poultry and fish more often than meat. When you do choose meat, choose only lean cuts and trim all visible fat.
- Remove the skin from poultry before cooking.
- Decrease or avoid high-fat processed luncheon meats and sausages.
- When preparing meat, fish, or poultry, avoid frying. Bake, roast, or broil them instead.
- Use margarine made from polyunsaturated oils like sunflower, safflower, corn, soybean, or cottonseed, rather than butter, lard, or shortening.
- Avoid foods that are high in palm kernel oil, palm oil, coconut oil, and cocoa butter by checking food labels. Ingredients are listed by weight—with the ingredients contained in the greatest amounts listed first and those contained in the least amounts listed last. A food that lists these types of oils first is high in saturated fat.

About This Counter

This counter lists the calorie (CAL), total fat (FAT), and cholesterol (CHOL) content of hundreds of common foods, including generic foods, brand name items, and fast foods. The individual food items are grouped into common categories, like "Beverages" and "Poultry," which are listed in alphabetical order. After the description of each item, a specific portion size is noted. The values for calories, total fat, and cholesterol are for the portion size listed. The total fat for each item is listed in

INTRODUCTION

grams (g) and the total cholesterol is listed in milligrams (mg).

Values in this counter were obtained from the United States Department of Agriculture and from food labels, manufacturers, and processors. While every effort has been made to ensure that these values are accurate and current at the time of printing, changes in values can occur at the time of food processing. Some food items have an "na" or a "tr" listed in one of the columns. The "na" means that the content was unavailable to us at the time of printing. The "tr" means that the food item contains only trace amounts of fat or cholesterol.

Baked Goods

FOOD/PORTION SIZE	CAL	FAT (g)	CHOL (mg)
CAKE			
Angelfood, enriched mix, tube cake, 1 piece (1/12 cake)	125	tr	0
Carrot, with cream cheese frosting, home recipe, 1 piece (1/16 cake)	385	21	74
Carrot, with cream cheese frosting, home recipe, whole 10-in. diameter tube cake	6,175	328	1,183
Cheesecake, 1 piece (1/12 cake)	280	18	170
Cheesecake, Jell-O, 8-in. cake, made with whole milk, 1/8 cake	280	13	30
Cheesecake, whole 9-in. diameter cake	3,350	213	2,053
Coffeecake, crumb, 1 piece (1/6 cake)	230	7	47
Coffeecake, crumb, 7 3/4 × 5 5/8 × 1 1/4-in. cake	1,385	41	279
Devil's food, with chocolate frosting, 1 2 1/2-in. cupcake	120	4	19
Devil's food, with chocolate frosting, 1 piece (1/16 cake)	235	8	37
Devil's food, with chocolate frosting, 2-layer cake	3,755	136	598
Fruitcake, dark, home recipe, 1 piece (1/32 cake)	165	7	20
Fruitcake, dark, home recipe, 7 1/2-in. tube cake	5,185	228	640
Gingerbread, 1 piece (1/9 cake)	175	4	1
Gingerbread, 8-in. square cake	1,575	39	6
Pound, 1 slice (1/17 loaf)	120	5	32
Pound, 8 1/2 × 3 1/2 × 3 1/4-in. loaf	2,025	94	555
Pound, commercial, 1 loaf	1,935	94	1,100
Pound, commercial, 1 slice (1/17 loaf)	110	5	64

BAKED GOODS

FOOD/PORTION SIZE	CAL	FAT (g)	CHOL (mg)
Sheet, plain, without frosting, 1 piece (1/9 cake)	315	12	61
Sheet, plain, without frosting, 9-in. square cake	2,830	108	552
Sheet, plain, with uncooked white frosting, 1 piece (1/9 cake)	445	14	70
Sheet, plain, with uncooked white frosting, 9-in. square cake	4,020	129	636
Snack, devil's food cream filled, 1 cake (2/pk)	105	4	15
Snack, sponge cream filled, 1 cake (2/pk)	155	5	7
White, with white frosting, commercial, 1 piece (1/16 cake)	260	9	3
White, with white frosting, commercial, 2-layer cake	4,170	148	46
Yellow, with chocolate frosting, commercial, 1 piece (1/16 cake)	245	11	38
Yellow, with chocolate frosting, commercial, 2-layer cake	3,895	175	609
Yellow, with chocolate frosting, enriched mix, 1 piece (1/16 cake)	235	8	36
Yellow, with chocolate frosting, enriched mix, 2-layer cake	3,735	125	576

COOKIES

Animal Crackers, Barnum's, 11 cookies	130	4	na
Chocolate chip, commercial, 4 cookies	180	9	5
Chocolate chip, home recipe, 4 cookies	185	11	18
Chocolate chip, refrigerated dough, 4 cookies	225	11	22

FOOD/PORTION SIZE	CAL	FAT (g)	CHOL (mg)
Oatmeal Chocolate Chip, Almost Home, 2 cookies	130	5	na
Oatmeal, with raisins, 4 cookies	245	10	2
Oreo, 3 cookies	140	6	na
Oreo, Double Stuff, 2 cookies	140	7	na
Peanut Butter Fudge, Almost Home, 2 cookies	140	7	na
Peanut butter, home recipe, 4 cookies	245	14	22
Sandwich (chocolate or vanilla), 4 cookies	195	8	0
Shortbread, commercial, 4 small cookies	155	8	27
Shortbread, home recipe, 2 large cookies	145	8	0
Shortbread, Lorna Doone, 4 cookies	140	7	na
Sugar, refrigerated dough, 4 cookies	235	12	29
Wafers, vanilla, 10 cookies	185	7	25

PASTRY

FOOD/PORTION SIZE	CAL	FAT (g)	CHOL (mg)
Danish, fruit, 4¼-in. round, 1 pastry	235	13	56
Danish, plain, 1 oz.	110	6	24
Danish, plain, 4¼-in. round, 1 pastry	220	12	49
Danish, plain, 12-oz. packaged ring, 1 ring	1,305	71	292
Toaster, 1 pastry	210	6	0

PIE

FOOD/PORTION SIZE	CAL	FAT (g)	CHOL (mg)
Apple, crust made with enriched flour and vegetable shortening, 1 piece (⅙ pie)	405	18	0
Apple, crust made with enriched flour and vegetable shortening, 9-in. pie	2,420	105	0

BAKED GOODS

FOOD/PORTION SIZE	CAL	FAT (g)	CHOL (mg)
Blueberry, crust made with enriched flour and vegetable shortening, 1 piece (1/6 pie)	380	17	0
Blueberry, crust made with enriched flour and vegetable shortening, 9-in. pie	2,285	102	0
Cherry, crust made with enriched flour and vegetable shortening, 1 piece (1/6 pie)	410	18	0
Cherry, crust made with enriched flour and vegetable shortening, 9-in. pie	2,465	107	0
Chocolate Mousse Pie, Jell-O, made with whole milk, 1/8 pie	250	15	30
Coconut Cream Pie, Jell-O, made with whole milk, 1/8 pie	260	17	30
Creme, crust made with enriched flour and vegetable shortening, 1 piece (1/6 pie)	455	23	8
Creme, crust made with enriched flour and vegetable shortening, 9-in. pie	2,710	139	46
Custard, crust made with enriched flour and vegetable shortening, 1 piece (1/6 pie)	330	17	169
Custard, crust made with enriched flour and vegetable shortening, 9-in. pie	1,985	101	1,010
Lemon meringue, crust made with enriched flour and vegetable shortening, 1 piece (1/6 pie)	355	14	143
Lemon meringue, crust made with enriched flour and vegetable shortening, 9-in. pie	2,140	86	857

FOOD/PORTION SIZE	CAL	FAT (g)	CHOL (mg)
Peach, crust made with enriched flour and vegetable shortening, 1 piece (1/6 pie)	405	17	0
Peach, crust made with enriched flour and vegetable shortening, 9-in. pie	2,410	101	0
Pecan, crust made with enriched flour and vegetable shortening, 1 piece (1/6 pie)	575	32	95
Pecan, crust made with enriched flour and vegetable shortening, 9-in. pie	3,450	189	569
Piecrust, home recipe, made with enriched flour and vegetable shortening, 9-in. shell	900	60	0
Piecrust, mix, 9-in., 2-crust pie	1,485	93	0
Pumpkin, crust made with enriched flour and vegetable shortening, 1 piece (1/6 pie)	320	17	109
Pumpkin, crust made with enriched flour and vegetable shortening, 9-in. pie	1,920	102	655

MISCELLANEOUS

FOOD/PORTION SIZE	CAL	FAT (g)	CHOL (mg)
Brownies, Fudge 'n Nut, Almost Home, 1 brownie	160	7	na
Brownies, with nuts and frosting, commercial, 1 brownie	100	4	14
Brownies, with nuts and frosting, home recipe, 1 brownie	95	6	18
Doughnuts, cake, plain, 1 doughnut	210	1	20
Doughnuts, yeast, glazed, 1 doughnut	235	13	21
Fig bars, square/rectangular, 4 cookies	210	4	27

Baking Products & Condiments

FOOD/PORTION SIZE	CAL	FAT (g)	CHOL (mg)
Bacos, 2 tsp.	25	1	0
Baking powder for home use, 1 tsp.	5	0	0
Baking soda for home use, 1 tsp.	5	0	0
Barbecue Sauce, Hickory Smoke Flavor, Kraft, 2 tbsp.	40	1	0
Barbecue Sauce, Hickory Smoke, Open Pit, 1 tbsp.	25	0	0
Barbecue Sauce, Hot, Kraft, 2 tbsp.	40	1	0
Barbecue Sauce, Hot 'n Tangy, Open Pit, 1 tbsp.	25	0	0
Barbecue Sauce, Italian Seasonings, Kraft, 2 tbsp.	45	1	0
Barbecue Sauce, Kansas City Style, 2 tbsp.	45	1	0
Barbecue Sauce, Kraft, 2 tbsp.	40	1	0
Barbecue Sauce, Mesquite 'n Tangy, Open Pit, 1 tbsp.	25	0	0
Barbecue Sauce, Mesquite Smoke, Kraft, 2 tbsp.	45	1	0
Barbecue Sauce, Onion Bits, Kraft, 2 tbsp.	50	1	0
Barbecue Sauce, Original, Open Pit, 1 tbsp.	25	0	0
Barbecue Sauce, Original with Minced Onions, Open Pit, 1 tbsp.	25	0	0
Barbecue Sauce, Sweet 'n Tangy, Open Pit, 1 tbsp.	25	0	0
Barbecue Sauce, Thick'n Spicy, Chunky, Kraft, 2 tbsp.	50	1	0

FOOD/PORTION SIZE	CAL	FAT (g)	CHOL (mg)
Barbecue Sauce, Thick'n Spicy Hickory Smoked, Kraft, 2 tbsp.	50	1	0
Barbecue Sauce, Thick'n Spicy Kansas City Style, Kraft, 2 tbsp.	60	1	0
Barbecue Sauce, Thick'n Spicy Original, Kraft, 2 tbsp.	50	1	0
Barbecue Sauce, Thick'n Spicy with Honey, Kraft, 2 tbsp.	60	1	0
Barbecue Sauce, Thick 'n Tangy Hickory, Open Pit, 1 tbsp.	25	0	0
Barley, pearled, light, uncooked, 1 cup	700	2	0
Bulgur, uncooked, 1 cup	600	3	0
Butterscotch Topping, Artificially Flavored, Kraft, 1 tbsp.	60	1	0
Caramel Topping, Kraft, 1 tbsp.	60	0	0
Catsup, 1 cup	290	1	0
Catsup, 1 tbsp.	15	tr	0
Catsup, Weight Watchers, 1 tbsp.	8	0	na
Celery seed, 1 tsp.	10	1	0
Chili powder, 1 tsp.	10	tr	0
Chocolate Caramel Topping, Kraft, 1 tbsp.	60	0	0
Chocolate Chips, Real, Semi-Sweet, Baker's, 1/4 cup	200	12	0
Chocolate Flavored Chips, Semi-Sweet, Baker's, 1/4 cup	190	9	0
Chocolate, German's Sweet Chocolate, Baker's, 1 oz.	140	10	0
Chocolate, Semi-Sweet, Baker's, 1 oz.	140	8	0
Chocolate Topping, Kraft, 1 tbsp.	50	0	0
Chocolate, Unsweetened, Baker's, 1 oz.	140	15	0
Cinnamon, 1 tsp.	5	tr	0
Cocktail Sauce, Sauceworks, 1 tbsp.	12	0	0

BAKING PRODUCTS & CONDIMENTS

FOOD/PORTION SIZE	CAL	FAT (g)	CHOL (mg)
Coconut, Angel Flake, Baker's, (bag) 1/3 cup	120	8	0
Coconut, Angel Flake, Baker's, (can) 1/3 cup	110	9	0
Coconut, Premium Shred, Baker's, 1/3 cup	140	9	0
Cornmeal, bolted, dry, 1 cup	440	4	0
Cornmeal, degermed, enriched, cooked, 1 cup	120	tr	0
Cornmeal, degermed, enriched, dry, 1 cup	500	2	0
Cornmeal, whole-ground, unbolted, dry, 1 cup	435	5	0
Curry powder, 1 tsp.	5	tr	0
Flour, buckwheat, light, sifted, 1 cup	340	1	0
Flour, cake/pastry, enriched, sifted, spooned, 1 cup	350	1	0
Flour, carob, 1 cup	255	tr	0
Flour, self-rising, enriched, unsifted, spooned, 1 cup	440	1	0
Flour, wheat, all-purpose, sifted, spooned, 1 cup	420	1	0
Flour, wheat, all-purpose, unsifted, spooned, 1 cup	455	1	0
Flour, whole-wheat from hard wheats, stirred, 1 cup	400	2	0
Garlic powder, 1 tsp.	10	tr	0
Honey, strained or extracted, 1 cup	1,030	0	0
Horseradish, Cream Style Prepared, Kraft, 1 tbsp.	8	0	0
Horseradish, Prepared, Kraft, 1 tbsp.	4	0	0
Horseradish Sauce, Kraft, 1 tbsp.	50	5	5
Horseradish Sauce, Sauceworks, 1 tbsp.	50	5	5
Hot Fudge Topping, Kraft, 1 tbsp.	70	3	0

FOOD/PORTION SIZE	CAL	FAT (g)	CHOL (mg)
Jams and preserves, 1 tbsp.	55	tr	0
Jellies, 1 tbsp.	50	tr	0
Marshmallow Creme, Kraft, 1 oz.	90	0	0
Mayonnaise, Hellman's, 1 tbsp.	100	11	5
Mayonnaise, imitation, 1 tbsp.	35	3	4
Mayonnaise, Light, Reduced Calorie, Kraft, 1 tbsp.	45	5	5
Mayonnaise, Real, Kraft, 1 tbsp.	100	12	5
Mayonnaise, regular, 1 tbsp.	100	11	8
Mustard, Dijon, Grey Poupon, 1 tbsp.	18	1	na
Mustard, Horseradish, Kraft, 1 tbsp.	4	0	0
Mustard, prepared yellow, 1 tsp. or individual packet	5	tr	0
Mustard, Pure Prepared, Kraft, 1 tbsp.	4	0	0
Mustard Sauce, Hot, Sauceworks, 1 tbsp.	35	2	5
Mustard, Spicy Brown, Gulden's, .25 oz.	8	0	na
Onion powder, 1 tsp.	5	tr	0
Oregano, 1 tsp.	5	tr	0
Paprika, 1 tsp.	5	tr	0
Pepper, black, 1 tsp.	5	tr	0
Pineapple Topping, Kraft, 1 tbsp.	50	0	0
Red Raspberry Topping, Kraft, 1 tbsp.	50	0	0
Relish, finely chopped sweet, 1 tbsp.	20	tr	0
Salad Dressing, Light, Miracle Whip, 1 tbsp.	45	4	5
Salad Dressing, Miracle Whip, 1 tbsp.	70	7	5
Salsa, Green Chile, Mild/Medium, Ortega, 1 oz.	8	0	na
Salsa, Green Chile, Hot, Ortega, 1 oz.	10	0	na
Salt, 1 tsp.	0	0	0

BAKING PRODUCTS & CONDIMENTS

FOOD/PORTION SIZE	CAL	FAT (g)	CHOL (mg)
Sandwich Spread, Kraft, 1 tbsp.	50	5	5
Shake 'N Bake Oven Fry Coating, Extra Crispy Recipe for Chicken, 1/4 pouch	110	2	0
Shake 'N Bake Oven Fry Coating, Extra Crispy Recipe for Pork, 1/4 pouch	120	3	0
Shake 'N Bake Oven Fry Coating, Homestyle Recipe for Chicken, 1/4 pouch	80	2	0
Shake 'N Bake Seasoning Mixture, Country Mild Recipe, 1/4 pouch	80	4	0
Shake 'N Bake Seasoning Mixture, Italian Herb Recipe, 1/4 pouch	80	1	0
Shake 'N Bake Seasoning Mixture, Original Barbecue Recipe for Chicken, 1/4 pouch	90	2	0
Shake 'N Bake Seasoning Mixture, Original Barbecue Recipe for Pork, 1/4 pouch	80	2	0
Shake 'N Bake Seasoning Mixture, Original Recipe for Chicken, 1/4 pouch	80	2	0
Shake 'N Bake Seasoning Mixture, Original Recipe for Fish, 1/4 pouch	70	1	0
Shake 'N Bake Seasoning Mixture, Original Recipe for Pork, 1/4 pouch	80	1	0
Steak Sauce, A.1., 1 tbsp.	12	0	na
Strawberry Topping, Kraft, 1 tbsp.	50	0	0
Sugar, brown, pressed down, 1 cup	820	0	0
Sugar, powdered, sifted, spooned into cup, 1 cup	385	0	0
Sugar, white, granulated, 1 cup	770	0	0

FOOD/PORTION SIZE	CAL	FAT (g)	CHOL (mg)
Sweet'n Sour Sauce, Sauceworks, 1 tbsp.	20	0	0
Syrup, chocolate-flavored syrup or topping, fudge type, 2 tbsp.	125	5	0
Syrup, chocolate-flavored syrup or topping, thin type, 2 tbsp.	85	tr	0
Syrup, molasses, cane, blackstrap, 2 tbsp.	85	0	0
Syrup, table syrup (corn & maple), 2 tbsp.	122	0	0
Tartar sauce, 1 tbsp.	75	8	4
Tartar Sauce, Hellman's, 1 tbsp.	70	8	5
Tartar Sauce, Kraft, 1 tbsp.	70	8	5
Tartar Sauce, Natural Lemon Herb Flavor, Sauceworks, 1 tbsp.	70	8	5
Tartar Sauce, Sauceworks, 1 tbsp.	70	8	5
Vinegar, cider, 1 tbsp.	tr	0	0
Walnut Topping, Kraft, 1 tbsp.	90	5	0
Yeast, baker's dry active, 1 package	20	tr	0
Yeast, brewer's dry, 1 tbsp.	25	tr	0

Beverages

FOOD/PORTION SIZE	CAL	FAT (g)	CHOL (mg)
ALCOHOL			
Beer, light, 12 fl. oz.	95	0	0
Beer, regular, 12 fl. oz.	150	0	0
Gin, rum, vodka, whiskey, 80-proof, 1¹/₂ fl. oz.	95	0	0
Gin, rum, vodka, whiskey, 86-proof, 1¹/₂ fl. oz.	105	0	0

BEVERAGES

FOOD/PORTION SIZE	CAL	FAT (g)	CHOL (mg)
Gin, rum, vodka, whiskey, 90-proof, 1½ fl. oz.	110	0	0
Wine, dessert, 3½ fl. oz.	140	0	0
Wine, table, red, 3½ fl. oz.	75	0	0
Wine, table, white, 3½ fl. oz.	80	0	0

BREAKFAST DRINKS

Carnation Instant Breakfast, Chocolate, 1 envelope	130	1	na
Carnation Instant Breakfast, Strawberry, 1 envelope	130	1	na
Carnation Instant Breakfast, Vanilla, 1 envelope	130	1	na
Tang Breakfast Beverage Crystals, 6 fl. oz.	90	0	0
Tang Sugar Free Breakfast Beverage Crystals, 6 fl. oz.	6	0	0

COFFEE

Brewed, 6 fl. oz.	tr	tr	0
Cafe Amaretto, General Foods International Coffees, 6 fl. oz.	50	2	0
Cafe Amaretto, General Foods Sugar Free International Coffees, 6 fl. oz.	35	3	0
Cafe Francais, General Foods International Coffees, 6 fl. oz.	50	3	0
Cafe Francais, General Foods Sugar Free International Coffees, 6 fl. oz.	35	2	0
Cafe Irish Cream, General Foods International Coffees, 6 fl. oz.	60	3	0
Cafe Irish Cream, General Foods Sugar Free International Coffees, 6 fl. oz.	30	2	0
Cafe Vienna, General Foods International Coffees, 6 fl. oz.	60	2	0

FOOD/PORTION SIZE	CAL	FAT (g)	CHOL (mg)
Cafe Vienna, General Foods Sugar Free International Coffees, 6 fl. oz.	30	2	0
Double Dutch Chocolate, General Foods International Coffees, 6 fl. oz.	50	2	0
Instant, prepared, 6 fl. oz.	tr	tr	0
Irish Mocha Mint, General Foods International Coffees, 6 fl. oz.	50	2	0
Irish Mocha Mint, General Foods Sugar Free International Coffees, 6 fl. oz.	25	2	0
Orange Capuccino, General Foods International Coffees, 6 fl. oz.	60	2	0
Orange Capuccino, General Foods Sugar Free International Coffees, 6 fl. oz.	30	2	0
Postum Coffee Flavor Instant Hot Beverage, 6 fl. oz.	12	0	0
Swiss Mocha, General Foods International Coffees, 6 fl. oz.	50	2	0
Swiss Mocha, General Foods Sugar Free International Coffees, 6 fl. oz.	30	2	0

JUICE

FOOD/PORTION SIZE	CAL	FAT (g)	CHOL (mg)
Apple, bottled or canned, 1 cup	115	tr	0
Apple/Cranberry, DelMonte Fruit Blends, 8.45 oz.	140	0	na
Cranberry juice cocktail, bottled, sweetened, 1 cup	145	tr	0
Cranberry Juice Cocktail, Ocean Spray, 6 oz.	110	0	na
Grape, canned or bottled, 1 cup	155	tr	0
Grape, frozen concentrate, sweetened, diluted, 1 cup	125	tr	0
Grape, frozen concentrate, sweetened, undiluted, 6-fl.-oz. can	385	1	0

BEVERAGES

FOOD/PORTION SIZE	CAL	FAT (g)	CHOL (mg)
Grapefruit, canned, sweetened, 1 cup	115	tr	0
Grapefruit, canned, unsweetened, 1 cup	95	tr	0
Grapefruit, frozen concentrate, unsweetened, diluted, 1 cup	100	tr	0
Grapefruit, frozen concentrate, unsweetened, undiluted, 6-oz. can	300	1	0
Grapefruit, Kraft Pure 100% Unsweetened, 6 oz.	70	0	0
Grapefruit, raw, 1 cup	95	tr	0
Lemon, canned or bottled, unsweetened, 1 cup	50	1	0
Lemon, canned or bottled, unsweetened, 1 tbsp.	5	tr	0
Lemon, frozen, single-strength, unsweetened, 6-oz. can	50	1	0
Lemon, raw, 1 cup	60	tr	0
Lime, canned, unsweetened, 1 cup	50	1	0
Lime, raw, 1 cup	65	tr	0
Orange and grapefruit, canned, 1 cup	105	tr	0
Orange, canned, unsweetened, 1 cup	105	tr	0
Orange, frozen concentrate, diluted, 1 cup	110	tr	0
Orange, frozen concentrate, undiluted, 6-oz. can	340	tr	0
Orange/Grapefruit, Kraft Pure 100% Unsweetened, 6 oz.	80	0	0
Orange, Kraft Pure 100% Unsweetened, 6 oz.	90	0	0
Orange/Pineapple, Kraft Pure 100% Unsweetened, 6 oz.	80	0	0
Orange, raw, 1 cup	110	tr	0
Pineapple/Orange, DelMonte Fruit Blends, 8.45 oz.	140	0	na

FOOD/PORTION SIZE	CAL	FAT (g)	CHOL (mg)
Pineapple, unsweetened, canned, 1 cup	140	tr	0
Prune, canned or bottled, 1 cup	180	tr	0
Tangerine, canned, sweetened, 1 cup	125	tr	0
V-8, 100% Vegetable, 6 oz.	35	0	na
V-8, Spicey Hot Vegetable, 6 oz.	35	0	na
Vegetable juice cocktail, canned, 1 cup	75	tr	0

MILK

FOOD/PORTION SIZE	CAL	FAT (g)	CHOL (mg)
Buttermilk, 1 cup	100	2	9
Buttermilk, dried, 1 cup	465	7	83
Canned, condensed, sweetened, 1 cup	980	27	104
Canned, evaporated, skim, 1 cup	200	1	9
Canned, evaporated, whole, 1 cup	340	19	74
Chocolate, lowfat (1%), 1 cup	160	3	7
Chocolate, lowfat (2%), 1 cup	180	5	17
Chocolate Malt Flavor, Ovaltine Classic, 3/4 oz.	80	0	0
Chocolate, regular, 1 cup	210	8	31
Cocoa Mix, Carnation, Milk Chocolate, 1 envelope	110	1	na
Cocoa Mix, Carnation, Rich Chocolate, 1 envelope	110	1	na
Cocoa Mix, Carnation, Rich Chocolate with Marshmallows, 1 envelope	110	1	na
Cocoa, powder, prepared with nonfat dry milk, 1 serving	100	1	1
Cocoa, powder, prepared with whole milk, 1 serving	225	9	33
Dried, nonfat, instant, 1 3.2-oz. envelope	325	1	17
Dried, nonfat, instant, 1 cup	245	tr	12
Eggnog (commercial), 1 cup	340	19	149

BEVERAGES

FOOD/PORTION SIZE	CAL	FAT (g)	CHOL (mg)
Fudge Drink, Slender Chocolate, 10 oz.	220	4	na
Lowfat (2%), milk solids added, 1 cup	105	2	10
Lowfat (2%), no milk solids, 1 cup	120	5	18
Malt Drink, Slender Chocolate, 10 oz.	220	4	na
Malted, chocolate, powder, 3/4 oz.	85	1	1
Malted, chocolate, powder, prepared, 1 serving	235	9	34
Malted Milk Chocolate, Kraft Instant, 3 tsp.	240	9	25
Malted, Natural, Kraft Instant, 3 tsp.	240	10	25
Malted, natural, powdered, 3/4 oz.	85	2	4
Malted, natural, powdered, prepared with milk, 1 serving	235	10	37
Malt Flavor, Ovaltine Classic, 3/4 oz.	80	0	0
Nonfat (skim), milk solids added, 1 cup	90	1	5
Nonfat (skim), no milk solids, 1 cup	85	tr	4
Shake Mix, Alba 77 Fit n' Frosty, Chocolate, 1 envelope	70	0	na
Shake Mix, Alba 77 Fit n' Frosty, Milk Chocolate, 1 envelope	70	0	na
Shake Mix, Alba 77 Fit n' Frosty, Strawberry, 1 envelope	70	0	na
Shake Mix, Alba 77 Fit n' Frosty, Vanilla, 1 envelope	70	0	na
Shakes, thick, chocolate, 10-oz. container	335	8	30
Shakes, thick, vanilla, 10-oz. container	315	9	33
Whole (3.3% fat), 1 cup	150	8	33

SOFT DRINKS, CARBONATED

	CAL	FAT	CHOL
7-Up, Diet, 6 oz.	2	0	na

FOOD/PORTION SIZE	CAL	FAT (g)	CHOL (mg)
7-Up, Diet, 6 oz.	2	0	na
7-Up, Diet Cherry, 6 oz.	2	0	na
Club Soda, Schweppes, 6 fl. oz.	0	0	0
Coca-Cola, 6 fl. oz.	77	0	0
Coca-Cola Classic, 6 fl. oz.	72	0	0
Coke, diet, 6 fl. oz.	0	0	na
Cola, regular, 12 fl. oz.	160	0	0
Diet-Rite, Black Cherry, 6 oz.	2	0	na
Diet-Rite, Cola, 6 oz.	2	0	na
Diet-Rite, Pink Grapefruit, 6 oz.	2	0	na
Diet-Rite, Red Raspberry, 6 oz.	2	0	na
Diet-Rite, Tangerine, 6 oz.	2	0	na
Dr. Pepper (Diet), 6 oz.	2	0	na
Fresca, 6 oz.	2	0	na
Ginger ale, 12 fl. oz.	125	0	0
Ginger Ale, Canada Dry, Diet, 6 oz.	2	0	na
Ginger Ale, Schweppes, Diet, 6 oz.	2	0	na
Grape, carbonated, 12 fl. oz.	180	0	0
Lemon-lime, carbonated, 12 fl. oz.	155	0	0
Orange, carbonated, 12 fl. oz.	180	0	0
Pepper type, carbonated, 12 fl. oz.	160	0	0
Pepsi Cola, Caffeine-Free, Diet, 6 oz.	0	0	na
Pepsi Cola, Diet, 6 oz.	0	0	na
Root beer, 12 fl. oz.	165	0	0
Root Beer, A & W, Diet, 6 oz.	2	0	na
Root Beer, Barrelhead, Diet, 6 oz.	2	0	na

SOFT DRINKS, NONCARBONATED

FOOD/PORTION SIZE	CAL	FAT (g)	CHOL (mg)
Country Time Drink Mix, Sugar Sweetened, Lemonade/Pink Lemonade, 8 fl. oz.	80	0	0
Country Time Drink Mix, Sugar Sweetened, Lemon-Lime, 8 fl. oz.	80	0	0

BEVERAGES

FOOD/PORTION SIZE	CAL	FAT (g)	CHOL (mg)
Country Time Sugar Free Drink Mix, Lemonade/Pink Lemonade, 8 fl. oz.	4	0	0
Country Time Sugar Free Drink Mix, Lemon-Lime, 8 fl. oz.	4	0	0
Crystal Light Sugar Free Drink Mix, all flavors, 8 fl. oz.	4	0	0
Fruit punch drink, noncarbonated, canned, 6 fl. oz.	85	0	0
Grape drink, noncarbonated, canned, 6 fl. oz.	100	0	0
Hi-C Cherry Drink, 6 oz.	100	0	na
Hi-C Citrus Cooler Drink, 6 oz.	100	0	na
Hi-C Double Fruit Cooler Drink, 6 oz.	90	0	na
Hi-C Fruit Punch Drink, 6 oz.	100	0	na
Hi-C Hula Punch Drink, 6 oz.	80	0	na
Kool-Aid Koolers Juice Drink, all flavors, 8.45 fl. oz.	130	0	0
Kool-Aid Soft Drink Mix Sugar-Sweetened, all flavors, 8 fl. oz.	80	0	0
Kool-Aid Soft Drink Mix Unsweetened, all flavors, 8 fl. oz.	2	0	0
Kool-Aid Soft Drink Mix Unsweetened, all flavors, with sugar added, 8 fl. oz.	100	0	0
Kool-Aid Sugar-Free Soft Drink Mix, all flavors, 8 fl. oz.	4	0	0
Lemonade concentrate, frozen, diluted, 6 fl. oz.	80	tr	0
Lemonade concentrate, frozen, undiluted, 6-fl.-oz. can	425	tr	0
Limeade concentrate, frozen, diluted, 6 fl. oz.	75	tr	0
Limeade concentrate, frozen, undiluted, 6-fl.-oz. can	410	tr	0

FOOD/PORTION SIZE	CAL	FAT (g)	CHOL (mg)
Ocean Spray, Cran-Apple Drink, 6 oz.	130	0	na
Ocean Spray, Cran-Grape Drink, 6 oz.	130	0	na
Ocean Spray, Cran-Raspberry Drink, 6 oz.	110	0	na
Pineapple-grapefruit juice drink, 6 fl. oz.	90	tr	0
Wylers, Bunch O'Berries Punch Mix, Sweetened, 8 oz.	90	0	na
Wylers, Bunch O'Berries Punch Mix, Unsweetened, 8 oz.	2	0	na
Wylers, Lemonade Drink Mix, Sweetened, 8 oz.	90	0	na
Wylers, Lemonade Drink Mix, Unsweetened, 8 oz.	4	0	na
Wylers, Tropical Punch Mix, Sweetened, 8 oz.	90	0	na
Wylers, Tropical Punch Mix, Unsweetened, 8 oz.	2	0	na
Wylers, Wild Cherry Mix, Sweetened, 8 oz.	90	0	na
Wylers, Wild Cherry Mix, Unsweetened, 8 oz.	2	0	na

TEA

FOOD/PORTION SIZE	CAL	FAT (g)	CHOL (mg)
Berry, Crystal Light Fruit-Tea Sugar Free Drink Mix, 8 fl. oz.	4	0	0
Brewed, 8 fl. oz.	tr	tr	0
Citrus, Crystal Light Fruit-Tea Sugar Free Drink Mix, 8 fl. oz.	4	0	0
Iced Tea, Crystal Light Sugar Free Drink Mix, 8 fl. oz.	4	0	0
Instant, powder, sweetened, 8 fl. oz.	85	tr	0
Instant, powder, unsweetened, 8 fl. oz.	tr	tr	0

BREADS & CEREALS

FOOD/PORTION SIZE	CAL	FAT (g)	CHOL (mg)
Natural Brew, Crystal Light Fruit-Tea Sugar Free Drink Mix, 8 fl. oz.	4	0	0
Tropical Fruit, Crystal Light Fruit-Tea Sugar Free Drink Mix, 8 fl. oz.	4	0	0

MISCELLANEOUS

Gatorade Lemon-Lime, 8.45 oz.	60	0	na
Gatorade Orange, 8.45 oz.	60	0	0
Postum Instant Hot Beverage, 6 fl. oz.	12	0	0

Breads & Cereals

FOOD/PORTION SIZE	CAL	FAT (g)	CHOL (mg)
BISCUITS			
Baking powder, home recipe, 1 biscuit	100	5	tr
Baking powder, mix, 1 biscuit	95	3	tr
Baking powder, refrigerated dough, 1 biscuit	65	2	1
BREAD			
Boston brown, canned, $3^1/_4 \times ^1/_2$-in. slice	95	1	3
Cracked-wheat, 1 slice	65	1	0
Crumbs, enriched, dry, grated, 1 cup	390	5	5
French, enriched, $5 \times 2^1/_2 \times 1$-in. slice	100	1	0

FOOD/PORTION SIZE	CAL	FAT (g)	CHOL (mg)
Italian, enriched, $4^{1}/_{2} \times 3^{1}/_{4} \times 3/_{4}$-in. slice	85	tr	0
Mixed grain, enriched, 1 slice	65	2	0
Oatmeal, enriched, 1 slice	65	1	0
Pita, enriched, white, $6^{1}/_{2}$-in. diameter, 1 pita	165	1	0
Pumpernickel, $2/_{3}$ rye, $1/_{3}$ wheat, 1 slice	80	1	0
Raisin, enriched, 1 slice,	65	1	0
Roman Meal, 1 slice	70	1	0
Rye, $2/_{3}$ wheat, $1/_{3}$ rye, $4^{3}/_{4} \times 3^{3}/_{4} \times 7/_{16}$-in. slice	65	1	0
Vienna, enriched, $4^{3}/_{4} \times 4 \times 1/_{2}$-in. slice	70	1	0
Wheat, enriched, 1 slice	65	1	0
Wheat, Home Pride, Buttertop, 1 slice	70	1	na
White, enriched, 1 slice	65	1	0
White, enriched, cubes, 1 cup	80	1	0
White, enriched, soft crumbs, 1 cup	120	2	0
White, Home Pride Buttertop, 1 slice	70	1	na
White, Wonder, 1 slice	70	1	0
Whole-wheat, 16-slice loaf, 1 slice	70	1	0

CEREALS, COLD

FOOD/PORTION SIZE	CAL	FAT (g)	CHOL (mg)
40% Bran Flakes, Kellogg's, 1 oz. ($3/_{4}$ cup)	90	1	0
40% Bran Flakes, Post, 1 oz. ($2/_{3}$ cup)	90	tr	0
100% Natural Cereal, 1 oz. ($1/_{4}$ cup)	135	6	tr
All-Bran, 1 oz. ($1/_{3}$ cup)	70	1	0
Alpha-Bits, 1 oz.	110	1	0
Alpha-Bits, with $1/_{2}$ cup whole milk, 1 oz.	190	5	15
Apple Cinnamon Natural, 1 oz.	126	4.9	na
Apple Jacks, 1 oz.	110	0	0

BREADS & CEREALS

FOOD/PORTION SIZE	CAL	FAT (g)	CHOL (mg)
Cap'n Crunch, 1 oz. (3/4 cup)	120	3	0
Cap'n Crunch Peanut Butter, 1 oz.	119	3.0	na
Cheerios, 1 oz. (1 1/4 cup)	110	2	0
Cheerios, Honey-Nut, 1 oz. (3/4 cup)	105	1	0
Cocoa Krispies, 1 oz.	110	0	0
Cocoa Pebbles, 1 oz.	110	1	0
Cocoa Pebbles, with 1/2 cup whole milk, 1 oz.	190	5	15
Cocoa Puffs, 1 oz.	110	1	0
Corn Chex, 1 oz.	110	0	0
Corn Flakes, Kellogg's, 1 oz. (1 1/4 cup)	110	tr	0
Corn Flakes, Toasties, 1 oz. (1 1/4 cup)	110	tr	0
Cracklin' Bran, 1 oz.	110	4	0
Crispy Wheats & Raisins, 1 oz.	110	1	0
Crunchy Bran, 1 oz.	89	1.3	na
Crunchy Nut Ohs, 1 oz.	127	4.2	na
C.W. Post Hearty Granola, 1 oz.	130	4	0
C.W. Post Hearty Granola, with 1/2 cup whole milk, 1 oz.	200	8	15
C.W. Post Hearty Granola with Raisins, 1 oz.	120	4	0
C.W. Post Hearty Granola with Raisins, with 1/2 cup whole milk, 1 oz.	200	8	15
Fortified Oat Flakes, 1 oz.	110	1	0
Fortified Oat Flakes, with 1/2 cup whole milk, 1 oz.	180	5	15
Froot Loops, 1 oz. (1 cup)	110	1	0
Frosted Mini-Wheats, 1 oz.	100	0	0
Fruit & Fibre-Dates, Raisins, Walnuts, 1 oz.	90	1	0
Fruit & Fibre-Dates, Raisins, Walnuts, with 1/2 cup whole milk, 1 oz.	160	5	15
Fruit & Fibre-Harvest Medley, 1 oz.	90	1	0

FOOD/PORTION SIZE	CAL	FAT (g)	CHOL (mg)
Fruit & Fibre-Harvest Medley, with ¹/₂ cup whole milk, 1 oz.	170	5	15
Fruit & Fibre-Mountain Trail, 1 oz.	90	1	0
Fruit & Fibre-Mountain Trail, with ¹/₂ cup whole milk, 1 oz.	170	5	15
Fruit & Fibre-Tropical Fruit, 1 oz.	90	1	0
Fruit & Fibre-Tropical Fruit, with ¹/₂ cup whole milk, 1 oz.	170	5	15
Fruity Pebbles, 1 oz.	110	1	0
Fruity Pebbles, with ¹/₂ cup whole milk, 1 oz.	190	5	15
Golden Grahams, 1 oz. (³/₄ cup)	110	1	tr
Grape-Nuts, 1 oz.	110	0	0
Grape-Nuts, with ¹/₂ cup whole milk, 1 oz.	180	4	15
Grape-Nuts Flakes, 1 oz.	100	1	0
Grape-Nuts Flakes, with ¹/₂ cup whole milk, 1 oz.	180	5	15
Grape-Nuts, Raisin, with ¹/₂ cup whole milk, 1 oz.	170	4	15
Honeycomb, 1 oz.	110	0	0
Honeycomb, with ¹/₂ cup whole milk, 1 oz.	190	4	15
Honey Graham Ohs, 1 oz.	122	3.2	na
Just Right Fiber Nuggets, 1 oz.	100	1	0
Just Right Fruit & Nuts, 1 oz.	140	1	0
Kix, 1 oz.	110	0	0
Life, 1 oz.	101	1.7	na
Life, Cinnamon, 1 oz.	101	1.7	na
Lucky Charms, 1 oz. (1 cup)	110	1	0
Malt-O-Meal, 1 cup	120	tr	0
Mueslix Five Grain, 1 oz.	140	1	0
Natural Bran Flakes, 1 oz.	90	0	0
Natural Bran Flakes, with ¹/₂ cup whole milk, 1 oz.	160	4	15
Natural Raisin Bran, Post, 1 oz.	80	0	0
Natural Raisin Bran, Post, with ¹/₂ cup whole milk, 1 oz.	160	4	15

BREADS & CEREALS

FOOD/PORTION SIZE	CAL	FAT (g)	CHOL (mg)
Nature Valley Granola, 1 oz. (1/3 cup)	125	5	0
Nutri Grain Almonds & Raisins, 1 oz.	140	2	0
Nutri Grain Biscuits, 1 oz.	90	0	0
Nutri Grain Wheat & Raisins, 1 oz.	130	0	0
Oat Squares, 1 oz.	105	1.6	na
Popeye Puffed Rice, 1/2 oz.	50	0	na
Popeye Puffed Wheat, 1/2 oz.	50	0	na
Popeye Sweet Crunch, 1 oz.	113	1.8	na
Post Toasties Corn Flakes, 1 oz.	110	0	0
Post Toasties Corn Flakes, with 1/2 cup whole milk, 1 oz.	180	4	15
Product 19, 1 oz. (3/4 cup)	110	tr	0
Puffed Rice, Quaker Oats, 0.50 oz.	54	0.1	0
Puffed Wheat, Quaker Oats, 0.50 oz.	50	0.2	0
Raisin Bran, Kellogg's, 1 oz. (3/4 cup)	90	1	0
Raisin Bran, Post, 1 oz. (1/2 cup)	85	1	0
Raisin Date Natural, 1 oz.	123	5	na
Rice Chex, 1 oz.	110	0	0
Rice Krispies, 1 oz. (1 cup)	110	tr	0
Shredded Wheat, 1 oz. (2/3 cup)	100	1	0
Shredded Wheat, Spoon Size, 1 oz.	90	na	na
Smurf-Berry Crunch, 1 oz.	110	1	0
Smurf-Berry Crunch, with 1/2 cup whole milk, 1 oz.	190	5	15
Special K, 1 oz. (1 1/3 cup)	110	tr	tr
Sugar Frosted Flakes, Kellogg's, 1 oz. (3/4 cup)	110	tr	0
Sugar Smacks, 1 oz. (3/4 cup)	105	1	0
Sun Country Granola with Almonds, 1 oz.	130	5.3	0
Sun Country Granola with Raisins, 1 oz.	125	4.8	0

FOOD/PORTION SIZE	CAL	FAT (g)	CHOL (mg)
Sun Country Granola with Raisins & Dates, 1 oz.	123	4.5	0
Super Golden Crisp, 1 oz.	110	0	0
Super Golden Crisp, with 1/2 cup whole milk, 1 oz.	180	4	15
Super Sugar Crisp, 1 oz. (7/8 cup)	105	tr	0
Total, 1 oz. (1 cup)	100	1	0
Total, Whole Wheat, 1 oz.	110	1	0
Trix, 1 oz. (1 cup)	110	tr	0
Wheat Chex, 1 oz.	100	0	0
Wheat Germ, Honey Crunch, Kretschmer, 1 oz.	105	2.8	0
Wheaties, 1 oz. (1 cup)	100	tr	0

CEREALS, HOT

FOOD/PORTION SIZE	CAL	FAT (g)	CHOL (mg)
Corn grits, instant, plain, 1 cup	80	tr	0
Corn grits, regular/quick, enriched, 1 cup	145	tr	0
Cream of Wheat, Mix 'n Eat, plain, 1 packet	100	tr	0
Cream of Wheat, regular/quick/instant, 1 cup	140	tr	0
Malt-O-Meal, Chocolate, 1 oz.	100	0	na
Malt-O-Meal, Quick, 1 oz.	100	0	na
Oatmeal/rolled oats, instant, fortified, flavored, 1 packet	160	2	0
Oatmeal/rolled oats, instant, fortified, plain, 1 packet	105	2	0
Oatmeal/rolled oats, regular/quick/instant, nonfortified, 1 cup	145	2	0
Oats, Instant, Apple Cinnamon, Quaker Oats, 1.25 oz.	118	1.5	0
Oats, Instant, Bananas & Cream, Quaker Oats, 1.25 oz.	131	2.3	0
Oats, Instant, Blueberries & Cream, Quaker Oats, 1.25 oz.	131	2.4	0
Oats, Instant, Cinnamon Spice, Quaker Oats, 1.63 oz.	164	2.1	0

BREADS & CEREALS

FOOD/PORTION SIZE	CAL	FAT (g)	CHOL (mg)
Oats, Instant, Maple & Brown Sugar, Quaker Oats, 1.50 oz.	152	2.1	0
Oats, Instant, Peaches & Cream, Quaker Oats, 1.25 oz.	129	2.2	0
Oats, Instant, Raisin Date Walnut, Quaker Oats, 1.30 oz.	141	3.8	0
Oats, Instant, Raisin Spice, Quaker Oats, 1.50 oz.	149	2	0
Oats, Instant, Regular, Quaker Oats, 1 oz.	94	2	0
Oats, Instant, Strawberries & Cream, Quaker Oats, 1.25 oz.	129	2	0
Oats, Old Fashioned, Quaker Oats, 1 oz.	99	2	0
Oats, Quick, Quaker Oats, 1 oz.	99	2	0
Wheateena, 1 oz.	100	na	na
Whole Wheat Hot Natural, Quaker Oats, 1 oz.	92	0.6	0

CRACKERS

Cheese, plain, 1-in. square, 10 crackers	50	3	6
Cheese, sandwich/peanut butter, 1 sandwich	40	2	1
Graham, plain, 2½-in. square, 2 crackers	60	1	0
Rye wafers, whole-grain, 2 wafers	55	1	0
Rykrisp, (Natural), ½	40	0	0
Rykrisp, (Sesame), ½	45	1	0
Saltines, 4 crackers	50	1	4
Snack-type, standard, 1 round cracker	15	1	0
Wheat, thin, 4 crackers	35	1	0
Whole-wheat wafers, 2 crackers	35	2	0

FOOD/PORTION SIZE	CAL	FAT (g)	CHOL (mg)
MELBA TOAST			
Garlic, Old London, 1/2 oz.	60	2	na
Onion, Old London, 1/2 oz.	60	2	na
Plain, 1 piece	20	tr	0
Rye, Old London, 1/2 oz.	60	2	na
Sesame, Old London, 1/2 oz.	60	2	na
MUFFINS			
Blueberry, home recipe, enriched flour, 1 muffin	135	5	19
Blueberry, mix, 1 muffin	140	5	45
Blueberry-Streusel Mix, Betty Crocker, 1 muffin	190	6	na
Bran, home recipe, enriched flour, 1 muffin	125	6	24
Bran, mix, 1 muffin	140	4	28
Corn, home recipe, enriched degermed cornmeal, 1 muffin	145	5	23
Corn, mix, 1 muffin	145	6	42
Corn, Mix, Dromedary, 1 muffin	120	4	na
English, Bays, 2 oz.	140	2	na
English, plain, enriched, 1 muffin	140	1	0
English, Wonder, 2 oz.	180	2	na
ROLLS			
Dinner, enriched commercial, 1 roll	85	2	tr
Dinner, home recipe, 1 roll	120	3	12
Frankfurter/hamburger, enriched commercial, 1 roll	115	2	tr
Hard, enriched commercial, 1 roll	155	2	tr
Hoagie/submarine, enriched commercial, 1 roll	400	8	tr
STUFFING MIX			
Americana New England, Stove Top, 1/2 cup	110	1	0

BREADS & CEREALS

FOOD/PORTION SIZE	CAL	FAT (g)	CHOL (mg)
Americana New England, Stove Top, prepared with butter, 1/2 cup	180	9	20
Americana San Francisco, Stove Top, 1/2 cup	110	1	0
Americana San Francisco, Stove Top, prepared with butter, 1/2 cup	170	9	20
Beef, Stove Top, 1/2 cup	110	1	0
Beef, Stove Top, prepared with butter, 1/2 cup	180	9	20
Chicken Flavor Bread, Quaker Oats Golden Grain, as prepared, 1 oz.	180	9	na
Chicken Flavor, Stove Top, prepared with butter, 1/2 cup	180	9	20
Chicken, Stove Top, 1/2 cup	110	1	0
Chicken, Stove Top Flexible Serving, 1/2 cup	120	3	0
Chicken, Stove Top Flexible Serving, prepared with butter, 1/2 cup	170	9	15
Cornbread Rice, Quaker Oats Golden Grain, as prepared, 1 oz.	180	9	na
Cornbread Rice, Quaker Oats Golden Grain, dry mix, 1 oz.	110	1	na
Cornbread, Stove Top, 1/2 cup	110	1	0
Cornbread, Stove Top Flexible Serving, 1/2 cup	120	3	0
Cornbread, Stove Top Flexible Serving, prepared with butter, 1/2 cup	170	8	15
Cornbread, Stove Top, prepared with butter, 1/2 cup	170	9	20
Country Style, Pepperidge Farm, 1 oz.	110	1	na
Enriched bread, dry, 1 cup	500	31	0
Enriched bread, moist, 1 cup	420	26	67

FOOD/PORTION SIZE	CAL	FAT (g)	CHOL (mg)
Herb Butter Wild Rice, Quaker Oats Golden Grain, as prepared, 1 oz.	180	9	na
Herb Butter Wild Rice, Quaker Oats Golden Grain, dry mix, 1 oz.	100	1	na
Herb, Pepperidge Farm, 1 oz.	110	1	na
Homestyle Herb, Stove Top Flexible Serving, 1/2 cup	120	3	0
Homestyle Herb, Stove Top Flexible Serving, prepared with butter, 1/2 cup	170	9	15
Long Grain and Wild Rice, Stove Top, 1/2 cup	120	1	0
Long Grain and Wild Rice, Stove Top, prepared with butter, 1/2 cup	180	9	20
Pork, Stove Top, 1/2 cup	110	1	0
Pork, Stove Top, prepared with butter, 1/2 cup	170	9	20
Savory Herbs, Stove Top, 1/2 cup	110	1	0
Savory Herbs, Stove Top, prepared with butter, 1/2 cup	180	9	20
Turkey, Stove Top, 1/2 cup	110	1	0
Turkey, Stove Top, prepared with butter, 1/2 cup	170	9	20
Wild Rice Bread, Quaker Oats Golden Grain, as prepared, 1 oz.	180	9	0.4
Wild Rice Bread, Quaker Oats Golden Grain, dry mix, 1 oz.	110	1	na
With Rice, Stove Top, 1/2 cup	110	1	0
With Rice, Stove Top, prepared with butter, 1/2 cup	180	9	20

MISCELLANEOUS

Bagel, plain, Lender's, 2 oz.	150	1	0
Bagel, plain/water, enriched, 1 bagel	200	2	0

FOOD/PORTION SIZE	CAL	FAT (g)	CHOL (mg)
Bran, unprocessed, Quaker Oats, 0.25 oz.	8	0.2	na
Croissant, with enriched flour, 1 croissant	235	12	13
Oat Bran, Quaker Oats, 1 oz.	92	2.1	0
Tortilla, corn, 1 tortilla	65	1	0
Wheat Bran, Kretschmer, 1 oz.	57	2.3	0
Wheat Germ, Kretschmer, 1 oz.	103	3.4	0

Candy

FOOD/PORTION SIZE	CAL	FAT (g)	CHOL (mg)
Baby Ruth, 1 oz.	130	6	na
Bonkers! (all flavors), 1 piece	20	0	na
Breath Savers (all flavors), 1 piece	8	0	na
Bubble Yum (all flavors), 1 piece	25	0	na
Bubble Yum, Sugarless (all flavors), 1 piece	20	0	na
Butterfinger, 1 oz.	130	6	na
Butter Mints, Kraft, 1 mint	8	0	0
Caramels, Kraft, 1 caramel	35	1	0
Caramels, plain or chocolate, 1 oz.	115	3	1
Care*Free Sugarless Gum (all flavors), 1 piece	8	0	na
Care*Free Sugarless Bubble Gum (all flavors), 1 piece	10	0	na
Charleston Chew! (all flavors), 1 oz.	120	3	na
Chocolate, bitter or baking, 1 oz.	145	15	0
Chocolate Fudgies, Kraft, 1 fudgie	35	1	0
Chocolate, milk, plain, 1 oz.	145	9	6

FOOD/PORTION SIZE	CAL	FAT (g)	CHOL (mg)
Chocolate, milk, with almonds, 1 oz.	150	10	5
Chocolate, milk, with peanuts, 1 oz.	155	11	5
Chocolate, milk, with rice cereal, 1 oz.	140	7	6
Chocolate, semi-sweet small pieces, 1 cup or 6 oz. (60/oz.)	860	61	0
Chocolate, sweet dark, 1 oz.	150	10	0
Fruit Stripe Gum/Bubble Gum (all flavors), 1 piece	10	0	na
Fudge, chocolate, plain, 1 oz.	115	3	1
Funmallows, Kraft, 1 marshmallow	25	0	0
Gum drops, 1 oz.	100	tr	0
Hard candy, 1 oz.	110	0	0
Jelly beans, 1 oz.	105	tr	0
Jet-Puffed Marshmallows, Kraft, 1 marshmallow	25	0	0
Kisses, Hershey, 9 pieces	220	13	na
Kit Kat, 1.12 oz.	175	9	na
Krackel, 1.65 oz.	250	14	na
Life Savers Roll Candy (all flavors), 1 piece	8	0	na
Marshmallows, 1 oz.	90	0	0
Milk Chocolate Bar, Hershey, 1 bar	220	12	0
Miniature Funmallows, Kraft, 10 marshmallows	18	0	0
Miniature Marshmallows, Kraft, 10 marshmallows	18	0	0
Mr. Goodbar, 1.85 oz.	300	20	na
Party Mints, Kraft, 1 mint	8	0	0
Peanut Brittle, Kraft, 1 oz.	140	5	0
Reese's Peanut Butter Cup, 2 cups	280	17	0
Rolo, 9 pieces	270	12	na
Skor, 1.4 oz.	220	14	na

FOOD/PORTION SIZE	CAL	FAT (g)	CHOL (mg)
Special Dark, Hershey, 1 bar	210	12	0
Sugar Babies, 1 pkg.	180	2	na
Sugar Daddy, 1 pop	150	1	na
Toffee, Kraft, 1 piece	30	1	0
Whatchamacallit, 1.8 oz.	270	15	na
Y&S Twizzlers, 1.0 oz.	100	1	na
Y&S Bites, 1.0 oz.	100	1	na

Cheese

FOOD/PORTION SIZE	CAL	FAT (g)	CHOL (mg)
American Flavored, Singles Pasteurized Process Cheese Product, Light n' Lively, 1 oz.	70	4	15
American Flavor, Imitation Pasteurized Process Cheese Food, Golden Image, 1 oz.	90	6	5
American Flavor, Pasteurized Process Cheese Product, Harvest Moon Brand, 1 oz.	70	4	15
American, pasteurized process cheese, 1 oz.	105	9	27
American, pasteurized process cheese food, 1 oz.	95	7	18
American, Pasteurized Process Cheese Loaf, Deluxe, 1 oz.	110	9	25
American, Pasteurized Process Cheese Slices, Deluxe, 1 oz.	110	9	25
American, pasteurized process cheese spread, 1 oz.	80	6	16
American, Pasteurized Process Cheese Spread, Kraft, 1 oz.	80	6	20
American, Process Cheese, Borden Lite-Line, 4 oz.	50	2	10

FOOD/PORTION SIZE	CAL	FAT (g)	CHOL (mg)
American, Sharp, Pasteurized Process Cheese Loaf, Old English, 1 oz.	110	9	30
American, Sharp, Pasteurized Process Slices, Old English, 1 oz.	110	9	30
American, Singles Pasteurized Process Cheese Food, Kraft, 1 oz.	90	7	20
American, Singles Pasteurized Process Cheese Food (white), Kraft, 1 oz.	90	7	20
Bleu, 1 oz.	100	8	21
Bleu, Natural, Kraft, 1 oz.	100	9	30
Brick, Natural, Kraft, 1 oz.	110	9	30
Camembert, 1 wedge (3 wedges/4-oz. container)	115	9	27
Caraway, Natural, Kraft, 1 oz.	100	8	30
Cheddar, 1-in. cube	70	6	18
Cheddar, 1 oz.	115	9	30
Cheddar, Extra Sharp, Cold Pack Cheese Food, Cracker Barrel, 1 oz.	90	7	20
Cheddar Flavored, Sharp, Singles Pasteurized Process Cheese Product, Light n' Lively, 1 oz.	70	4	15
Cheddar, Mild, Imitation, Golden Image, 1 oz.	110	9	5
Cheddar, Natural, Kraft, 1 oz.	110	9	30
Cheddar, Port Wine, Cheese Log with Almonds, Cracker Barrel, 1 oz.	90	6	15
Cheddar, Port Wine, Cold Pack Cheese Food, Cracker Barrel, 1 oz.	90	7	20
Cheddar, Sharp, Cheese Ball with Almonds, Cracker Barrel, 1 oz.	90	6	15

CHEESE

FOOD/PORTION SIZE	CAL	FAT (g)	CHOL (mg)
Cheddar, Sharp, Cheese Log with Almonds, Cracker Barrel, 1 oz.	90	6	15
Cheddar, Sharp, Cold Pack Cheese Food, Cracker Barrel, 1 oz.	90	7	20
Cheddar, Sharp, Process Cheese, Borden Lite-Line, 4 oz.	50	2	10
Cheddar, shredded, 1 cup	455	37	119
Cheddar, Smokey, Cheese Log with Almonds, Cracker Barrel, 1 oz.	90	6	15
Cheese Food, Cold Pack with Real Bacon, Cracker Barrel, 1 oz.	90	7	20
Cheese Food, Pasteurized Process Sharp Singles, Kraft, 1 oz.	100	8	25
Cheese Food, Pasteurized Process, Smokelle, 1 oz.	100	7	20
Cheese Food with Bacon, Pasteurized Process, Kraft, 1 oz.	90	7	20
Cheese Food with Garlic, Pasteurized Process, Kraft, 1 oz.	90	7	20
Cheese Spread with Bacon, Pasteurized Process, Kraft, 1 oz.	80	7	20
Cheese Spread, Hot Mexican, Pasteurized Process, Velveeta, 1 oz.	80	6	20
Cheese Spread, Mild Mexican, Pasteurized Process, Velveeta, 1 oz.	80	6	20
Cheese Spread, Pasteurized Process, Velveeta, 1 oz.	80	6	20
Cheese Spread, Sharp, Pasteurized Process, Old English, 1 oz.	90	7	20

FOOD/PORTION SIZE	CAL	FAT (g)	CHOL (mg)
Cheese Spread, Slices, Pasteurized Process, Velveeta, 1 oz.	90	6	20
Cheese Spread with Bacon, Pasteurized Process, Kraft, 1 oz.	90	7	20
Cheese Spread with Bacon, Sharp, Pasteurized Process, Squeez-A-Snak, 1 oz.	90	7	20
Cheese Spread with Garlic, Pasteurized Process, Kraft, 1 oz.	80	6	15
Cheese Spread with Pimentos, Pasteurized Process, Squeez-A-Snak, 1 oz.	90	7	20
Cheez Whiz, Hot Mexican, Pasteurized Process Cheese Spread, 1 oz.	80	6	15
Cheez Whiz, Mild Mexican, Pasteurized Process Cheese Spread, 1 oz.	80	6	15
Cheez Whiz, Pasteurized Process Cheese Spread, 1 oz.	80	6	20
Cheez Whiz, Pimento, Pasteurized Process Cheese Spread, 1 oz.	80	6	15
Cheez Whiz with Jalapeño Pepper, Pasteurized Process Cheese Spread, 1 oz.	80	6	15
Colby, Imitation, Golden Image, 1 oz.	110	9	5
Colby, Natural, Kraft, 1 oz.	110	9	30
Cottage, Breakstone Low-Fat, 4 oz.	90	3	na
Cottage, creamed, large curd, 1 cup	235	10	34
Cottage, creamed, small curd, 1 cup	215	9	31
Cottage, creamed, with fruit, 1 cup	280	8	25
Cottage, Lite n' Lively, 4 oz.	80	1	15
Cottage, low-fat (2%), 1 cup	205	4	19

CHEESE

FOOD/PORTION SIZE	CAL	FAT (g)	CHOL (mg)
Cottage, uncreamed, dry curd, 1 cup	125	1	10
Cream cheese, 1 oz.	100	10	31
Cream Cheese, Philadelphia Brand, 1 oz.	100	10	30
Cream Cheese Product, Pasteurized Process, Light Philadelphia Brand, 1 oz.	60	5	15
Cream Cheese, Soft Philadelphia Brand, 1 oz.	100	10	30
Cream Cheese, Whipped, Philadelphia Brand, 1 oz.	100	10	30
Cream Cheese, Whipped, with Bacon and Horseradish, Philadelphia Brand, 1 oz.	90	9	20
Cream Cheese, Whipped, with Bleu Cheese, Philadelphia Brand, 1 oz.	100	9	25
Cream Cheese, Whipped, with Chives, Philadelphia Brand, 1 oz.	90	9	25
Cream Cheese, Whipped, with Onions, Philadelphia Brand, 1 oz.	90	8	20
Cream Cheese, Whipped, with Pimentos, Philadelphia Brand, 1 oz.	90	9	25
Cream Cheese, Whipped, with Smoked Salmon, Philadelphia Brand, 1 oz.	100	9	25
Cream Cheese with Chives & Onion, Soft Philadelphia Brand, 1 oz.	100	9	30
Cream Cheese with Chives, Philadelphia Brand, 1 oz.	90	9	30
Cream Cheese with Honey, Soft Philadelphia Brand, 1 oz.	100	8	25
Cream Cheese with Olives & Pimento, Soft Philadelphia Brand, 1 oz.	90	8	30

FOOD/PORTION SIZE	CAL	FAT (g)	CHOL (mg)
Cream Cheese with Pimentos, Philadelphia Brand, 1 oz.	90	9	30
Cream Cheese with Pineapple, Soft Philadelphia Brand, 1 oz.	90	8	25
Cream Cheese with Smoked Salmon, Soft Philadelphia Brand, 1 oz.	90	8	25
Cream Cheese with Strawberries, Soft Philadelphia Brand, 1 oz.	90	8	25
Edam, Natural, Kraft, 1 oz.	90	7	20
Feta, 1 oz.	75	6	25
Garlic Flavor Pasteurized Process Cheese Spread, Squeez-A-Snak, 1 oz.	90	7	20
Gouda, Natural, Kraft, 1 oz.	110	9	30
Havarti, Casino, 1 oz.	120	11	35
Hickory Smoke Flavor, Pasteurized Process Cheese Spread, Squeez-A-Snak, 1 oz.	80	7	20
Jalapeño, Pasteurized Process Cheese Spread, Kraft, 1 oz.	80	6	20
Jalapeño Pepper Spread, Kraft, 1 oz.	70	5	15
Jalapeño, Singles Pasteurized Process Cheese Food, Kraft, 1 oz.	90	7	25
Light, Low-Cholesterol, Dorman's, 4 oz.	70	5	3
Limburger, Natural, Little Gem Size, Mohawk Valley, 1 oz.	90	8	25
Limburger, Pasteurized Process Cheese Spread, Mohawk Valley, 1 oz.	70	6	20
Monterey Jack, Natural, Kraft, 1 oz.	110	9	30
Monterey Jack, Natural, with Jalapeño Peppers, Kraft, 1 oz.	110	9	30
Monterey Jack, Natural, with Peppers, Mild, Kraft, 1 oz.	110	9	30

CHEESE

FOOD/PORTION SIZE	CAL	FAT (g)	CHOL (mg)
Monterey Jack, Singles Pasteurized Process Cheese Food, Kraft, 1 oz.	90	7	25
Mozzarella, Low Moisture, Casino, 1 oz.	90	7	25
Mozzarella, Part-Skim, Low Moisture, Kraft, 1 oz.	80	5	15
Mozzarella, made with part-skim milk, 1 oz.	80	5	15
Mozzarella, made with whole milk, 1 oz.	80	6	22
Mozzarella String with Jalapeño Pepper, Part-Skim, Low Moisture, Kraft, 1 oz.	80	5	20
Muenster, 1 oz.	105	9	27
Muenster, Natural, Kraft, 1 oz.	110	9	30
Neufchatel, Natural, Kraft, 1 oz.	80	7	25
Olives & Pimento Spread, Kraft, 1 oz.	70	5	15
Parmesan, grated, 1 cup	455	30	79
Parmesan, grated, 1 oz.	130	9	22
Parmesan, grated, 1 tbsp.	25	2	4
Parmesan, Grated, Kraft, 1 oz.	130	9	30
Parmesan, Natural, Kraft, 1 oz.	110	7	20
Peanut Butter 'n Cheese, Handi-Snacks Crackers, 1 package	190	13	0
Pimento Cheese Spread, Pasteurized Process, Velveeta, 1 oz.	80	6	20
Pimento, Pasteurized Process Cheese Slices, Deluxe, 1 oz.	100	8	25
Pimento, Singles Pasteurized Process Cheese Food, Kraft, 1 oz.	90	7	20
Pimento Spread, Kraft, 1 oz.	70	5	15
Pineapple Spread, Kraft, 1 oz.	70	5	15
Pizza Topping with Vegetable Oil, Lunch Wagon, 1 oz.	80	6	0

FOOD/PORTION SIZE	CAL	FAT (g)	CHOL (mg)
Provolone, 1 oz.	100	8	20
Provolone, Natural, Kraft, 1 oz.	100	7	25
Ricotta, made with part-skim milk, 1 cup	340	19	76
Ricotta, made with whole milk, 1 cup	430	32	124
Romano, Grated, Kraft, 1 oz.	130	9	30
Romano, Natural, Casino, 1 oz.	100	7	30
Sandwich Slices with Vegetable Oil, Lunch Wagon, 1 oz.	80	6	5
Scamorze, Part-Skim, Low Moisture, Kraft, 1 oz.	80	5	15
Swiss, 1 oz.	105	8	26
Swiss Flavored, Singles Pasteurized Process Cheese Product, Light n' Lively, 1 oz.	70	4	15
Swiss Flavor, Process Cheese, Borden Lite-Line, 4 oz.	50	2	10
Swiss, Light, No Salt, Dorman's, 4 oz.	100	8	na
Swiss, Natural, Aged, Kraft, 1 oz.	110	8	25
Swiss, Natural, Kraft, 1 oz.	110	8	25
Swiss, pasteurized process cheese, 1 oz.	95	7	24
Swiss, Pasteurized Process Cheese Slices, Deluxe, 1 oz.	90	7	25
Swiss, Singles Pasteurized Process Cheese Food, Kraft, 1 oz.	90	7	25

Creamers & Cream Substitutes

FOOD/PORTION SIZE	CAL	FAT (g)	CHOL (mg)
Coffee Rich, 1/2 oz.	20	2	0
Cool Whip Extra Creamy Dairy Recipe Whipped Topping, Birds Eye, 1 tbsp.	16	1	0
Cool Whip Non-Dairy Whipped Topping, Birds Eye, 1 tbsp.	12	1	0
Creamer, sweet, imitation, liquid, 1 tbsp.	20	1	0
Creamer, sweet, imitation, powdered, 1 tbsp.	10	1	0
Creamer, sour, 1 cup	495	48	102
Cream, sour, 1 tbsp.	25	3	5
Cream Substitute, Milnot, 1/2 cup	150	8	0
Cream, sweet, half-and-half, 1 cup	315	28	89
Cream, sweet, half-and-half, 1 tbsp.	20	2	6
Cream, sweet, light/coffee/table, 1 cup	470	46	159
Cream, sweet, light/coffee/table, 1 tbsp.	30	3	10
Cream, sweet, whipping, unwhipped, heavy, 1 cup	820	88	326
Cream, sweet, whipping, unwhipped, heavy, 1 tbsp.	50	6	21
Cream, sweet, whipping, unwhipped, light, 1 cup	700	74	265
Cream, sweet, whipping, unwhipped, light, 1 tbsp.	45	5	17
Cream Topping, Real, Kraft, 1/4 cup	25	2	10
Cream, whipped topping, pressurized, 1 cup	155	13	46

FOOD/PORTION SIZE	CAL	FAT (g)	CHOL (mg)
Cream, whipped topping, pressurized, 1 tbsp.	10	1	2
Sour dressing, filled cream-type, imitation, 1 cup	415	39	13
Sour dressing, filled cream-type, imitation, 1 tbsp.	20	2	1
Whipped Topping, Kraft, 1/4 cup	35	3	0
Whipped Topping Mix, Dream Whip, prepared with whole milk, 1 tbsp.	10	0	0
Whipped Topping Mix, Reduced Calorie, D-Zerta, 1 tbsp.	8	1	0
Whipped topping, sweet, imitation, frozen, 1 cup	240	19	0
Whipped topping, sweet, imitation, frozen, 1 tbsp.	15	1	0
Whipped topping, sweet, imitation, pressurized, 1 cup	185	16	0
Whipped topping, sweet, imitation, pressurized, 1 tbsp.	10	1	0
Whipped topping, sweet, powdered, prepared with whole milk, 1 cup	150	10	8
Whipped topping, sweet, powdered, prepared with whole milk, 1 tbsp.	10	tr	tr

Eggs

FOOD/PORTION SIZE	CAL	FAT (g)	CHOL (mg)
Egg Substitute, Scramblers, 4 oz.	60	3	0
Large, fried in butter, 1 egg	95	7	278
Large, hard-cooked, shell removed, 1 egg	80	6	274

FOOD/PORTION SIZE	CAL	FAT (g)	CHOL (mg)
Large, poached, 1 egg	80	6	273
Large, raw, white only, 1 white	15	tr	0
Large, raw, whole, without shell, 1 egg	80	6	274
Large, raw, yolk only, 1 yolk	65	6	272
Omelet, with milk, cooked in butter, 1 egg	110	8	282
Scrambled, with milk, cooked in butter, 1 egg	110	8	282

Fast Foods

FOOD/PORTION SIZE	CAL	FAT (g)	CHOL (mg)
ARBY'S			
Apple Turnover, 1 turnover	303	18.3	0
Bac'n Cheddar Deluxe, 1 sandwich	526	36.5	83
Beef 'N Cheddar, 1 sandwich	455	26.8	63
Cherry Turnover, 1 turnover	280	17.8	0
Chicken Breast Sandwich, 1 sandwich	509	29.1	83
Fish Fillet Sandwich, 1 sandwich	580	31.9	70
French Fries, 1 order (2.5 oz.)	215	9.7	8
Hot Ham 'N Cheese, 1 sandwich	292	13.7	45
Roast Beef, Junior, 1 sandwich	218	8.5	20
Roast Beef, King, 1 sandwich	467	19.2	49
Philly Beef 'N Swiss, 1 sandwich	460	28.4	107
Potato Cakes, 2 cakes (3 oz.)	201	12.9	13
Roast Beef, Giant, 1 sandwich	531	23.1	65
Roast Beef, Regular, 1 sandwich	353	14.8	39
Roast Beef, Super, 1 sandwich	501	22.1	40
Shake, Chocolate, 1 shake (12 oz.)	451	11.6	36

FOOD/PORTION SIZE	CAL	FAT (g)	CHOL (mg)
Shake, Jamocha, 1 shake (11.5 oz.)	368	10.5	35
Shake, Vanilla, 1 shake (11 oz.)	330	11.5	32
Turkey Deluxe, 1 sandwich	375	16.6	39

BURGER KING

FOOD/PORTION SIZE	CAL	FAT (g)	CHOL (mg)
Apple Pie, 1 pie	na	12	4
Breakfast Croissan'wich, 1 sandwich	304	19	243
Breakfast Croissan'wich with Bacon, 1 sandwich	355	24	249
Breakfast Croissan'wich with Ham, 1 sandwich	335	20	261
Breakfast Croissan'wich with Sausage, 1 sandwich	538	41	293
Cheeseburger, 1 cheeseburger	317	15	48
Cheeseburger, Bacon Double, 1 cheeseburger	510	31	104
Chicken Specialty Sandwich, 1 sandwich	688	40	82
French Fries, lightly salted, Regular	227	13	14
French Toast Sticks, 1 order	499	29	74
Great Danish, 1 pastry	500	36	6
Hamburger, 1 hamburger	275	12	37
Ham & Cheese Specialty Sandwich, 1 sandwich	471	27	77
Onion Rings, 1 order	274	16	0
Salad Dressing, 1000 Island, 1 serving	117	12	17
Salad Dressing, Bleu Cheese, 1 serving	156	16	22
Salad Dressing, House, 1 serving	130	13	11
Salad Dressing, Reduced Calorie Italian, 1 serving	14	1	0
Salad, without dressing, 1 salad	28	0	0
Scrambled Egg Platter, 1 platter	468	30	370
Scrambled Egg Platter with Bacon, 1 platter	536	36	378

FAST FOODS

FOOD/PORTION SIZE	CAL	FAT (g)	CHOL (mg)
Scrambled Egg Platter with Sausage, 1 platter	702	52	420
Whaler Fish Sandwich, 1 sandwich	488	27	77
Whopper, 1 sandwich	628	36	90
Whopper with Cheese, 1 sandwich	711	43	113
Whopper Jr., 1 sandwich	322	17	41
Whopper Jr. with Cheese, 1 sandwich	364	20	52

DAIRY QUEEN

Chicken Breast Fillet, 1 sandwich	608	34	78
Chicken Breast Fillet with Cheese, 1 sandwich	661	38	87
"Chipper" Sandwich, 1 sandwich	318	7	13
Cone, Chocolate, "Queen's Choice," 1 cone	326	16	52
Cone, Vanilla, "Queen's Choice," 1 cone	322	16	52
Fish Fillet, 1 sandwich	430	18	40
Fish Fillet with Cheese, 1 sandwich	483	22	49
"Fudge Nut Bar," 1 bar	406	25	10
"Heath" "Blizzard," 16 oz.	800	24	65
Hounder, 1 sandwich	480	36	80
Hounder with Chili, 1 sandwich	575	41	89
Malt, large, 21 oz.	889	21	60
Shake, large, 21 oz.	831	22	60

DOMINO'S

Pizza, Cheese, 2 slices	376	10.0	18.5
Pizza, Deluxe, 2 slices	498	20.4	39.8
Pizza, Double Cheese/Pepperoni, 2 slices	545	25.3	47.7
Pizza, Ham, 2 slices	417	11.0	26.0
Pizza, Pepperoni, 2 slices	460	17.5	28.0

CONSUMER GUIDE®

FOOD/PORTION SIZE	CAL	FAT (g)	CHOL (mg)
Pizza, Sausage/Mushroom, 2 slices	430	15.8	28.1
Pizza, Veggie, 2 slices	498	18.5	36.5

JACK IN THE BOX

FOOD/PORTION SIZE	CAL	FAT (g)	CHOL (mg)
Burger, Ham & Swiss, 1 hamburger	754	49	106
Burger, Monterey, 1 hamburger	865	57	152
Burger, Mushroom, 1 hamburger	470	24	64
Burger, Swiss and Bacon, 1 hamburger	681	47	92
Cheeseburger, 1 cheeseburger	325	17	41
Cheeseburger, Bacon, 1 cheeseburger	667	39	85
Cheesecake, 1 serving	309	17.5	63
Chicken Strip Dinner, 1 serving	689	30	100
Chicken Supreme, 1 sandwich	575	36	62
Crescent, Canadian, 1 serving	452	31	226
Crescent, Sausage, 1 serving	584	43	187
Crescent, Supreme, 1 serving	547	40	178
Dressing, Bleu Cheese, 1 serving	131	11	9.1
Dressing, Buttermilk House, 1 serving	181	18	10.3
Dressing, French, Reduced Calorie, 1 serving	80	4	0
Dressing, Thousand Island, 1 serving	156	15	11.4
Egg Platter, Scrambled, 1 serving	720	44	260
French Fries, large	353	19	13
French Fries, regular	221	12	8
Hamburger, 1 hamburger	288	13	26
Hot Apple Turnover, 1 serving	410	24	15
Jack, Breakfast, 1 serving	307	13	203
Jack, Jumbo, 1 serving	573	34	73
Jack, Jumbo, with Cheese, 1 serving	665	40	102
Jack, Moby, 1 serving	444	25	47
Nachos, Cheese, 1 serving	571	35	37
Nachos, Supreme, 1 serving	639	36	37

FAST FOODS

FOOD/PORTION SIZE	CAL	FAT (g)	CHOL (mg)
Onion Rings, 1 serving	382	23	27
Pancake Platter, 1 serving	630	27	85
Pita Club, without sauce, 1 serving	277	8	43
Pizza Pocket, 1 serving	497	28	32
Salad, Chef, 1 salad	295	18	107
Salad, Pasta & Seafood, 1 salad	394	22	48
Salad, Side, 1 salad	51	3	na
Salad, Taco, 1 salad	377	24	102
Sauce, BBQ, 1 serving	78	<1	0
Sauce, Mayo-Mustard, 1 serving	124	13	10
Sauce, Mayo-Onion, 1 serving	143	15	20
Sauce, Seafood Cocktail, 1 serving	57	<1	0
Shake, Chocolate Milk, 1 serving	330	7	25
Shake, Strawberry Milk, 1 serving	320	7	25
Shake, Vanilla Milk, 1 serving	320	6	25
Shrimp Dinner, 1 serving	731	37	157
Sirloin Steak Dinner, 1 serving	699	27	75
Taco, 1 serving	191	11	21
Taco, Super, 1 serving	288	17	37

McDONALD'S

FOOD/PORTION SIZE	CAL	FAT (g)	CHOL (mg)
Bacon Bits, 1 serving (3g)	16	1.2	0
Big Mac, 1 sandwich	562	32.4	103
Biscuit with Bacon, Egg, and Cheese, 1 biscuit	449	27.1	336
Biscuit with Biscuit Spread, 1 biscuit	260	12.7	1
Biscuit with Sausage, 1 biscuit	440	29.1	49
Biscuit with Sausage and Egg, 1 biscuit	529	35.3	358
Cheeseburger, 1 sandwich	308	13.8	53
Chicken McNuggets, 1 serving (113g)	288	16.3	65
Chow Mein Noodles, 1 serving (9g)	45	2.21	2
Cookies, Chocolaty Chip, 1 box	325	15.6	4
Cookies, McDonaldland, 1 box	288	9.2	0

FOOD/PORTION SIZE	CAL	FAT (g)	CHOL (mg)
Cone, Soft Serve, 1 cone	144	4.5	16
Croutons, 1 serving (11g)	52	2.17	0
Danish, Apple, 1 danish	369	17.9	25
Danish, Cinnamon Raisin, 1 danish	445	21	34
Danish, Iced Cheese, 1 danish	395	21.8	47
Danish, Raspberry, 1 danish	414	15.9	26
Dressing, 1000 Island, 1 packet	390	7.5	8
Dressing, Bleu Cheese, 1 packet	345	6.9	6
Dressing, French, 1 packet	232	5.2	0
Dressing, Lite Vinaigrette, 1 packet	60	.5	0
Dressing, Oriental, 1 packet	96	.1	0
Dressing, Ranch, 1 packet	332	8.6	5
Egg McMuffin, 1 sandwich	293	11.9	299
Eggs, Scrambled, 1 serving (100g)	157	11.1	545
Filet-o-Fish, 1 sandwich	442	26.1	50
French Fries, large	312	16.3	12
French Fries, regular	220	11.5	9
Hamburger, 1 hamburger	257	9.5	37
Hashbrowns, 1 serving (53g)	131	7.3	9
Honey, 1 serving (14g)	46	0	0
Hotcakes, with butter and syrup, 1 serving (176g)	413	9.2	21
McD.L.T., 1 sandwich	674	42.1	112
Muffin, English, with butter, 1 muffin	169	4.6	9
Pie, Apple, 1 pie	262	14.8	6
Quarter Pounder, 1 sandwich	414	20.7	86
Quarter Pounder with Cheese, 1 sandwich	517	29.2	118
Salad, Chef, 1 salad	231	13.6	152
Salad, Chicken, Oriental, 1 salad	141	3.4	78
Salad, Garden, 1 salad	112	6.8	107
Salad, Shrimp, 1 salad	104	2.8	193
Salad, Side, 1 salad	57	3.4	53
Sauce, Barbeque, 1 serving (32g)	53	0.5	0
Sauce, Hot Mustard, 1 serving (30g)	66	3.6	5

FAST FOODS

FOOD/PORTION SIZE	CAL	FAT (g)	CHOL (mg)
Sauce, Sweet-n-Sour, 1 serving (32g)	57	0.2	0
Sausage McMuffin, 1 serving	372	21.9	64
Sausage McMuffin with Egg, 1 serving	451	27.4	336
Sausage, Pork, 1 serving	180	16.3	48
Shake, Chocolate Milk,1 shake	388	10.6	41
Shake, Strawberry Milk, 1 shake	384	10.1	41
Shake, Vanilla Milk, 1 shake	354	10.2	41
Sundae, Hot Caramel, 1 sundae	343	9.1	35
Sundae, Hot Fudge, 1 sundae	313	9.4	28
Sundae, Strawberry, 1 sundae	283	7.3	27

TACO BELL

FOOD/PORTION SIZE	CAL	FAT (g)	CHOL (mg)
Bellbeefer, 1 serving	312.1	13.6	56.1
Burrito, Bean, 1 serving	359.6	10.9	13.8
Burrito, Bean, Green, 1 serving	353.9	10.9	58.7
Burrito, Beef, 1 serving	402.1	17.3	58.7
Burrito, Beef, Green, 1 serving	396.5	17.3	58.7
Burrito, Combo, 1 serving	380.9	14.1	36.2
Burrito, Combo, Green, 1 serving	375.2	14.1	36.2
Burrito, Double Beef, Supreme, 1 serving	464.5	22.8	58.7
Burrito, Double Beef, Supreme, Green, 1 serving	458.8	22.8	58.7
Burrito Supreme, 1 serving	422	18.8	35.4
Burrito Supreme, Green, 1 serving	416.3	18.8	35.4
Burrito Supreme Platter, 1 serving	773.7	36.9	79
Burrito Supreme Platter, Green, 1 serving	762.3	37	79
Cheesearito, 1 serving	311.9	12.8	29.2
Crispas, Cinnamon, 1 serving	266.1	15.9	1.8
Dressing, Ranch, 1 serving	235.6	24.8	35.5
Enchirito, 1 serving	381.8	20.1	38.6
Enchirito, Green, 1 serving	370.5	20.1	56.1
Fajita Steak Taco, 1 serving	235.4	10.9	14.3

FOOD/PORTION SIZE	CAL	FAT (g)	CHOL (mg)
Fajita Steak Taco with Guacamole, 1 serving	269.4	13.1	14.3
Fajita Steak Taco with Sour Cream, 1 serving	281.1	15.4	14.3
Jalapeño Peppers, 1 serving (100g)	20	.18	.8
Nachos, 1 serving	356.3	19.2	8.6
Pintos & Cheese, 1 serving	194.2	9.5	18.7
Pintos & Cheese, Green, 1 serving	188.6	9.5	18.7
Nachos Bellgrande, 1 serving	719.4	40.7	42.8
Pizza, Mexican, 1 serving	713.9	47.9	80.8
Salad, Seafood, without dressing, 1 serving	648.3	41.5	81.6
Salad, Seafood, without dressing/shell, 1 serving	216.8	11.4	81
Salad, Taco, without beans, 1 serving	821.8	57.2	80.5
Salad, Taco, without salsa, 1 serving	931.3	62	85.5
Salad, Taco, without shell, 1 serving	524.6	32.1	82.3
Salad, Taco, with Ranch Dressing, 1 serving	1,167.3	86.9	121
Salad, Taco, with Salsa, 1 serving	949.4	62.1	85.5
Salsa, 1 serving (90.7g)	18.1	.09	na
Sauce, Hot Taco, 1 packet,	2.5	.09	na
Sauce, Taco, 1 packet	2.06	.01	na
Taco, 1 serving	183.9	10.9	31.8
Taco Bellgrande, 1 serving	350.5	21.7	55.2
Taco Bellgrande Platter, 1 serving	1,001.5	50.8	80.2
Taco Bellgrande Platter, Green, 1 serving	990.2	50.8	80.2
Taco Light, 1 serving	411.2	28.9	57.3
Taco Light Platter, Green, 1 serving	1,050.9	58.1	82.2
Taco, Soft, 1 serving	228.3	11.8	31.8
Tostada, 1 serving	243.2	10.9	17.9
Tostada, Beefy, 1 serving	322.4	19.6	40.3

FAST FOODS

FOOD/PORTION SIZE	CAL	FAT (g)	CHOL (mg)
Tostada, Beefy, Green, 1 serving	316.5	19.6	40.3
Tostada, Green, 1 serving	237.5	10.9	17.8

WENDY'S

FOOD/PORTION SIZE	CAL	FAT (g)	CHOL (mg)
Big Classic, with Kaiser Bun, 1 sandwich	470	25	80
Biscuit, Buttermilk, 1 biscuit	320	17	tr
Bun, Kaiser, 1 bun	180	2	5
Bun, Multi-Grain, 1 bun	140	3	tr
Bun, White, 1 bun	140	2	tr
Cheese, American, 1 slice	60	6	15
Chicken Breast Filet, 1 sandwich	200	10	60
Chicken Fried Steak, 1 serving	580	41	95
Chicken Nuggets, Crispy, cooked in animal/vegetable oil, 6 pieces	290	21	55
Chicken Nuggets, Crispy, cooked in vegetable oil, 6 pieces	310	21	50
Chili, New, 1 serving	230	9	50
Chili, Regular, 1 serving	240	8	25
Condiments, Pre-Packaged, black pepper, 1 packet	0	0	0
Condiments, Pre-Packaged, creamer, nondairy, 3/8 oz.	14	1	0
Condiments, Pre-Packaged, half & half, 3/8 oz.	14	1	5
Condiments, Pre-Packaged, hot chili seasoning, 1 packet	6	na	na
Condiments, Pre-Packaged, ketchup, 1 packet	12	na	0
Cookie, Chocolate Chip, 1 cookie	320	17	5
Corn Relish, Old Fashion, 1/4 cup	35	na	na
Danish, Apple, 1 pastry	360	14	na
Danish, Cheese, 1 pastry	430	21	na
Danish, Cinnamon Raisin, 1 pastry	410	18	na
Dressing, Blue Cheese, 1 tbsp.	60	7	10
Dressing, Celery Seed, 1 tbsp.	70	6	5
Dressing, French, 1 tbsp.	70	6	0

FOOD/PORTION SIZE	CAL	FAT (g)	CHOL (mg)
Dressing, French Style, 1 tbsp.	70	5	0
Dressing, Golden Italian, 1 tbsp.	50	4	0
Dressing, Oil, 1 tbsp.	120	14	0
Dressing, Ranch, 1 tbsp.	50	6	5
Dressing, Reduced Calorie Bacon/Tomato, 1 tbsp.	45	4	tr
Dressing, Reduced Calorie Creamy Cucumber, 1 tbsp.	50	5	tr
Dressing, Reduced Calorie Italian, 1 tbsp.	25	2	0
Dressing, Reduced Calorie Thousand Island, 1 tbsp.	45	4	5
Dressing, Thousand Island, 1 tbsp.	70	7	5
Dressing, Wine Vinegar, 1 tbsp.	2	na	0
Egg, Fried, 1 egg	90	6	230
Eggs, Scrambled, 2 eggs	190	12	450
Fish Fillet, 1 serving	210	11	45
French Toast, 2 slices	400	19	115
Fries, cooked in animal/vegetable oil, regular	310	15	15
Fries, cooked in vegetable oil, regular	300	15	5
Frosty Dairy Dessert, small	400	14	50
Gravy, Sausage, 6 oz.	440	36	85
Hamburger, 1/4-lb. Single Patty	210	14	75
Hamburger, Kid's Meal, with White Bun, 1 hamburger	200	9	35
Omelet #1, Eggs, Ham, Cheese, 1 serving	290	21	355
Omelet #2, Eggs, Ham, Cheese, Mushrooms, 1 serving	250	17	450
Omelet #3, Eggs, Ham, Cheese, Onion, Green Pepper, 1 serving	280	19	525
Omelet #4, Eggs, Mushrooms, Green Pepper, Onion, 1 serving	210	15	460
Nuggets Sauce, Barbeque, 1 packet	50	na	0
Nuggets Sauce, Honey, 1 packet	45	na	0

FAST FOODS

FOOD/PORTION SIZE	CAL	FAT (g)	CHOL (mg)
Nuggets Sauce, Sweet Mustard, 1 packet	50	1	0
Nuggets Sauce, Sweet & Sour, 1 packet	45	na	0
Potato, Hot Stuffed Baked, Bacon & Cheese, 1 serving	570	30	22
Potato, Hot Stuffed Baked, Broccoli & Cheese, 1 serving	500	25	22
Potato, Hot Stuffed Baked, Cheese, 1 serving	590	34	22
Potato, Hot Stuffed Baked, Chili & Cheese, 1 serving	510	20	22
Potato, Hot Stuffed Baked, plain, 1 serving	250	2	tr
Potato, Hot Stuffed Baked, Sour Cream & Chives, 1 serving	460	24	15
Potatoes, Breakfast, 1 serving	360	22	20
Pudding, Butterscotch, 1/4 cup	90	4	tr
Salad, Chef (take-out), 1 salad	180	9	120
Salad, Garden (take-out), 1 salad	102	5	0
Salad, Taco, 1 salad	660	37	35
Sandwich, Breakfast, 1 sandwich	370	19	200
Sauce, Special, 1 tbsp.	40	3	5
Sauce, Taco, 1 packet	10	na	0
Sauce, Tartar, 1 tbsp.	90	na	10
Sausage Patty, 1 patty	200	18	45
Topping, Apple, 1 packet	130	na	0
Topping, Blueberry, 1 packet	60	na	0
Topping, Imitation Sour, 1 oz.	45	4	0

Fats & Oils

FOOD/PORTION SIZE	CAL	FAT (g)	CHOL (mg)
Butter Buds, 1 g	4	0	0
Butter, 1 pat	35	4	11
Butter, stick, 1/2 cup	810	92	247
Butter, 1 tbsp. (1/8 stick)	100	11	31
Lard, 1 cup	1,850	205	195
Lard, 1 tbsp.	115	13	12
Margarine, imitation, soft, 1 tbsp.	5	5	0
Margarine, Parkay, 1 tbsp.	100	11	0
Margarine, regular, hard, 1/2 cup (1 stick)	810	91	0
Margarine, regular, hard, 1 pat	35	4	0
Margarine, regular, hard, 1 tbsp. (1/8 stick)	100	11	0
Margarine, regular, soft, 1 tbsp.	100	11	0
Margarine, Soft Diet Parkay Reduced Calorie, 1 tbsp.	50	6	0
Margarine, Soft Parkay, 1 tbsp.	100	11	0
Margarine, Soft Parkay Corn Oil, 1 tbsp.	100	11	0
Margarine, Squeeze Parkay, 1 tbsp.	100	11	0
Margarine, spread, hard, 1/2 cup (1 stick)	610	69	0
Margarine, spread, hard, 1 pat	25	3	0
Margarine, spread, hard, 1 tbsp. (1/8 stick)	75	9	0
Margarine, spread, soft, 1 tbsp.	75	9	0
Margarine, Stick, Corn Oil, Mazola, 1 tbsp.	100	11	0
Margarine, Stick, Soy Oil, Chiffon, 1 tbsp.	100	11	0
Margarine, Stick, Soy Oil, Land O' Lakes, 1 tbsp.	97	4	0
Margarine, Stick, Soy Oil, Weight Watchers Reduced-Calorie, 1 tbsp.	*60*	*7*	*0*

FATS & OILS

FOOD/PORTION SIZE	CAL	FAT (g)	CHOL (mg)
Margarine, Stick, Sunflower Oil, Promise, 1 tbsp.	90	10	0
Margarine, Tub, Soy Oil, Chiffon, 1 tbsp.	90	10	0
Margarine, Tub, Soy Oil, Land O' Lakes, 1 tbsp.	97	4	0
Margarine, Tub, Soy Oil, Weight Watchers Reduced Calorie, 1 tbsp.	50	6	0
Margarine, Tub, Sunflower Oil, Promise, 1 tbsp.	90	10	0
Margarine, Whipped, Cup, Parkay, 1 tbsp.	60	7	0
Margarine, Whipped, Miracle Brand, 1 tbsp.	60	7	0
Margarine, Whipped, Stick, Miracle Brand, 1 tbsp.	70	7	0
Margarine, Whipped, Stick, Parkay, 1 tbsp.	60	7	0
Mayonnaise, *see* BAKING PRODUCTS & CONDIMENTS			
Oil, Corn, Mazola, 1 tbsp.	120	14	0
Oil, salad or cooking, corn, 1 cup	1,925	218	0
Oil, salad or cooking, corn, 1 tbsp.	125	14	0
Oil, salad or cooking, olive, 1 cup	1,910	216	0
Oil, salad or cooking, olive, 1 tbsp.	125	14	0
Oil, salad or cooking, peanut, 1 cup	1,910	216	0
Oil, salad or cooking, peanut, 1 tbsp.	125	14	0
Oil, salad or cooking, safflower, 1 cup	1,925	218	0
Oil, salad or cooking, safflower, 1 tbsp.	125	14	0
Oil, salad or cooking, soybean, hydrogenated, 1 cup	1,925	218	0
Oil, salad or cooking, sunflower, 1 cup	1,925	218	0

CONSUMER GUIDE®

FOOD/PORTION SIZE	CAL	FAT (g)	CHOL (mg)
Oil, salad or cooking, sunflower, 1 tbsp.	125	14	0
Oil, soybean-cottonseed blend, hydrogenated, 1 cup	1,925	218	0
Oil, salad or cooking, soybean, hydrogenated, 1 tbsp.	125	14	0
Oil, soybean-cottonseed blend, hydrogenated, 1 tbsp.	125	14	0
Oil, Sunflower, Sunlite, 1 tbsp.	120	14	0
Oil, Vegetable, Crisco, 1 tbsp.	120	14	0
Oil, Vegetable, Puritan, 1 tbsp.	120	14	0
Oil, Vegetable, Wesson, 1 tbsp.	120	14	0
Shortening, cooking, vegetable, 1 cup	1,810	205	0
Shortening, cooking, vegetable, 1 tbsp.	115	13	0
Shortening, Vegetable, Crisco, 1 tbsp.	110	12	0
Spray, Cooking (Vegetable), Pam, 1.25 seconds	7	1	0
Spray, No-Stick (Vegetable), Mazola, 2.5 seconds	6	1	0
Spread, 50% Fat, Parkay, 1 tbsp.	60	7	0
Spread, Cup, Kraft, 1 tbsp.	50	6	0
Spread, Light, Corn Oil, Parkay, 1 tbsp.	70	8	0
Spread, Stick, Kraft, 1 tbsp.	60	7	0
Spread, Tub (Vegetable), Shedd's, 1 tbsp.	70	7	0

Fish & Shellfish

FOOD/PORTION SIZE	CAL	FAT (g)	CHOL (mg)
Clams, canned, drained solids, 3 oz.	85	2	54
Clams, raw, meat only, 3 oz.	65	1	43
Crabmeat, canned, 1 cup	135	3	135
Fish sticks, frozen, reheated, 4 × 1 × 1/2-in. stick	70	3	26
Flounder, baked, with lemon juice, with butter, 3 oz.	120	6	68
Flounder, baked, with lemon juice, with margarine, 3 oz.	120	6	55
Flounder, baked, with lemon juice, without added fat, 3 oz.	80	1	59
Haddock, breaded, fried, 3 oz.	175	9	75
Halibut, broiled, with butter, with lemon juice, 3 oz.	140	6	62
Herring, pickled, 3 oz.	190	13	85
Oysters, breaded, fried, 1 oyster	90	5	35
Oysters, raw, meat only, 1 cup	160	4	120
Perch, ocean, breaded, fried, 1 fillet	185	11	66
Salmon, baked, red, 3 oz.	140	5	60
Salmon, canned, pink, solids and liquid, 3 oz.	120	5	34
Salmon, Pink, Bumble Bee, 3.5 oz.	160	8	na
Salmon, Red, Bumble Bee, 3.5 oz.	180	10	na
Salmon, smoked, 3 oz.	150	8	51
Sardines, canned in oil, drained, 3 oz.	175	9	85
Sardines, (in Vegetable Oil), King Oscar, 3.75 oz.	460	42	na
Scallops, breaded, frozen, reheated, 6 scallops	195	10	70
Shrimp, canned, drained solids, 3 oz.	100	1	128

FOOD/PORTION SIZE	CAL	FAT (g)	CHOL (mg)
Shrimp, French fried, 3 oz. (7 medium)	200	10	168
Sole, baked, with lemon juice, with butter, 3 oz.	120	6	68
Sole, baked, with lemon juice, with margarine, 3 oz.	120	6	55
Sole, baked, with lemon juice, without added fat, 3 oz.	80	1	59
Trout, broiled with butter and lemon juice, 3 oz.	175	9	71
Tuna, Albacore, Chunk (in Water), Starkist, 2 oz.	70	1	na
Tuna, Albacore (in Water), Bumble Bee, 2 oz.	60	1	na
Tuna, Albacore (in Water), Chicken of the Sea, 1 cup	490	32	na
Tuna, canned, drained solids, oil packed, chunk light, 3 oz.	165	7	55
Tuna, canned, drained solids, water packed, solid white, 3 oz.	135	1	48
Tuna, Chunk Light (in Vegetable Oil), Bumble Bee, 2 oz.	160	12	na
Tuna, Chunk Light, (in Vegetable Oil), Chicken of the Sea, 2 oz.	170	13	na
Tuna, Chunk Light (in Vegetable Oil), Starkist, 2 oz.	150	13	na
Tuna, Chunk Light (in Water), Bumble Bee, 2 oz.	60	1	na
Tuna, Chunk Light (in Water), Chicken of the Sea, 2 oz.	60	1	na
Tuna, Chunk Light (in Water), Starkist, 2 oz.	65	1	na
Tuna salad, 1 cup	375	19	80

Frozen Appetizers & Entrees

FOOD/PORTION SIZE	CAL	FAT (g)	CHOL (mg)
APPETIZERS			
Swanson's, Chicken Nuggets Platter, 8³/₄ oz.	460	25	na
Weaver, Chicken Mini Drums, 3 oz.	210	12	na
Weaver, Chicken Nuggets, 3 oz.	170	9	na
Weight Watchers, Baked Cheese Ravioli, 9 oz.	300	12	na
Weight Watchers, Chicken Nuggets, 3 oz.	180	10	na
COMBINATION ENTREES			
Swanson's, Mexican Style Combination Dinner, 14¹/₄ oz.	500	25	na
MEAT ENTREES			
La Choy, Fresh & Lite, Beef & Broccoli, 11 oz.	290	7	na
Lean Cuisine, Oriental Beef, 8⁵/₈ oz.	270	5	na
Lean Cuisine, Salisbury Steak, 9¹/₂ oz.	270	13	na
Swanson's, Salisbury Steak Dinner, 10³/₄ oz.	410	18	na
Swanson's, Veal Parmigiana, 12¹/₄ oz.	450	22	na
Weight Watchers, Lasagna with Meat Sauce, 11 oz.	330	13	na

FOOD/PORTION SIZE	CAL	FAT (g)	CHOL (mg)
POULTRY ENTREES			
La Choy, Fresh & Lite, Chicken Chow Mein, 11 oz.	270	9	na
La Choy, Fresh & Lite, Sweet & Sour Chicken, 10 oz.	280	4	na
Lean Cuisine, Breast of Chicken Marsala, 8⅛ oz.	190	5	na
Lean Cuisine, Chicken Cacciatore, 10⅞ oz.	280	10	na
Swanson's, Turkey White Meat Dinner, 11½ oz.	360	11	na
Weaver, Chicken Italian Style, 3 oz.	205	11	na
Weight Watchers, Chicken a la King, 9 oz.	220	7	na
Weight Watchers, Chicken Burritos, 5 oz.	300	11	na
SEAFOOD ENTREES			
Booth, Light Entree, Filet of Cod Au Gratin, 9½ oz.	280	11	na
Booth, Light Entree, Filet of Cod Mushroom, 9½ oz.	280	11	na
Booth, Light Entree, Shrimp Fettucine Alfredo, 10 oz.	260	8	na
Booth, Light Entree, Shrimp Oriental, 10 oz.	190	3	na
Booth, Light Entree, Shrimp New Orleans, 10 oz.	230	5	na
Lean Cuisine, Filet of Fish Divan, 12⅜ oz.	270	9	na
Lean Cuisine, Tuna Lasagna, 9¾ oz.	280	10	na
La Choy, Fresh & Lite, Shrimp with Lobster Sauce, 10 oz.	210	7	na
Mrs. Pauls, Light Entree, Fish Dijon, 8.75 oz.	220	9	na

FROZEN DESSERTS

FOOD/PORTION SIZE	CAL	FAT (g)	CHOL (mg)
Mrs. Pauls, Light Entree, Fish Mornay, 9 oz.	250	10	na
Mrs. Pauls, Light Entree, Shrimp Primavera, 9.5 oz.	190	4	na
Weight Watchers, Seafood Linguini, 9 oz.	220	7	na

Frozen Desserts

FOOD/PORTION SIZE	CAL	FAT (g)	CHOL (mg)
DAIRY			
Ice Cream, Butter Pecan, Breyers, 1 cup	150	8	na
Ice Cream, Chocolate, Breyers, 1 cup	160	8	na
Ice Cream, Chocolate, Sealtest, 1/2 cup	140	7	na
Ice Cream, Peach, Natural, Breyers, 1 cup	140	12	na
Ice Cream, Strawberry, Natural, Breyers, 1 cup	130	6	na
Ice Cream, Vanilla/Chocolate/ Strawberry, Sealtest, 1/2 cup	140	6	na
Ice Cream, Vanilla, Natural, Breyers, 1 cup	180	12	na
Ice cream, vanilla, regular, hardened, 1 cup	270	14	59
Ice cream, vanilla, rich, hardened, 1 cup	350	24	88
Ice Cream, Vanilla, Sealtest, 1/2 cup	140	7	na
Ice cream, vanilla, soft serve, 1 cup	375	23	153

FOOD/PORTION SIZE	CAL	FAT (g)	CHOL (mg)
Ice Milk, Chocolate, Weight Watchers, ¹/₂ cup	100	3	na
Ice Milk, Neapolitan, Weight Watchers, ¹/₂ cup	100	3	na
Ice milk, vanilla, hardened, 1 cup	185	6	18
Ice milk, vanilla, soft serve, 1 cup	225	5	13
Ice milk, Vanilla, Weight Watchers, ¹/₂ cup	100	3	na
Sherbet, 1 cup	270	4	14

SPECIALTY BARS

	CAL	FAT (g)	CHOL (mg)
Fruit Bars, all flavors, Jell-O, 1 bar	45	0	0
Fruit n' Juice Bars, Pineapple, Dole, 1 bar	70	1	na
Fruit n' Juice Bars, Raspberry-Pineapple, Dole Freshlites, 1 bar	25	1	na
Gelatin Pops, all flavors, Jell-O, 1 bar	35	0	0
Popsicle, 3-fl.-oz. size, 1 popsicle	70	0	0
Pudding Pops, Chocolate-Caramel Swirl, Jell-O, 1 bar	80	2	0
Pudding Pops, Chocolate-Covered Chocolate, Jell-O, 1 bar	130	7	0
Pudding Pops, Chocolate-Covered Vanilla, Jell-O, 1 bar	130	7	0
Pudding Pops, Chocolate, Jell-O, 1 bar	80	2	0
Pudding Pops, Chocolate-Vanilla Swirl, Jell-O, 1 bar	70	2	0
Pudding Pops, Chocolate with Chocolate Chips, Jell-O, 1 bar	80	3	0
Pudding Pops, Vanilla, Jell-O, 1 bar	70	2	0
Pudding Pops, Vanilla with Chocolate Chips, Jell-O, 1 bar	80	3	0

Fruit

FOOD/PORTION SIZE	CAL	FAT (g)	CHOL (mg)
Applesauce, canned, sweetened, 1 cup	195	tr	0
Applesauce, canned, unsweetened, 1 cup	105	tr	0
Apples, dried, sulfured, 10 rings	155	tr	0
Apples, raw, peeled, sliced, 1 cup	65	tr	0
Apples, raw, unpeeled, 3¼-in. diameter, 1 apple	125	1	0
Apricot nectar, canned, 1 cup	140	tr	0
Apricots, canned, heavy syrup pack, 3 halves	70	tr	0
Apricots, canned, juice pack, 3 halves	40	tr	0
Apricots, dried, cooked, unsweetened, 1 cup	210	tr	0
Apricots, dried, uncooked, 1 cup	310	1	0
Apricots, raw, 3 apricots	50	tr	0
Avocados, California, raw, whole, 1 avocado	305	30	0
Avocados, Florida, raw, whole, 1 avocado	340	27	0
Bananas, raw without peel, whole, 1 banana	105	1	0
Blackberries, raw, 1 cup	75	1	0
Blueberries, frozen, sweetened, 10 oz.	230	tr	0
Blueberries, raw, 1 cup	80	1	0
Cantaloupe, raw, ½ melon	95	1	0
Cherries, sour, red, pitted, canned, waterpack, 1 cup	90	tr	0
Cherries, sweet, raw, 10 cherries	50	1	0
Cranberry sauce, sweetened, canned, strained, 1 cup	420	tr	0
Dates, chopped, 1 cup	490	1	0
Dates, whole, without pits, 10 dates	230	tr	0

FOOD/PORTION SIZE	CAL	FAT (g)	CHOL (mg)
Figs, dried, 10 figs	475	2	0
Fruit cocktail, canned, heavy syrup, 1 cup	185	tr	0
Fruit cocktail, canned, juice pack, 1 cup	115	tr	0
Fruit Cocktail, DelMonte, 1/2 cup	80	0	na
Fruit Cocktail, DelMonte Lite, 1/2 cup	50	0	na
Fruit Cocktail, Libby's Lite, 1/2 cup	50	0	na
Fruit, Mixed, Chunky, Lite, Libby's, 1/2 cup	50	0	na
Fruit, Mixed, in Syrup, Birds Eye Quick Thaw Pouch, 5 oz.	120	0	0
Fruit Salad, Kraft Pure Chilled, 1/2 cup	50	0	0
Grapefruit, canned, with syrup, 1 cup	150	tr	0
Grapefruit, raw, 1/2 grapefruit	40	tr	0
Grapefruit Sections, Kraft, Pure, Chilled Unsweetened, 1/2 cup	50	0	0
Grapes, Thompson seedless, 10 grapes	35	tr	0
Grapes, Tokay/Emperor, seeded, 10 grapes	40	tr	0
Honeydew melon, raw, 1/10 melon	45	tr	0
Kiwifruit, raw, without skin, 1 kiwifruit	45	tr	0
Lemons, raw, without peel and seeds, 1 lemon	15	tr	0
Mangos, raw, 1 mango	135	1	0
Nectarines, raw, 1 nectarine	65	1	0
Olives, canned, green, 4 medium or 3 extra large	15	2	0
Olives, ripe, mission, pitted, 3 small or 2 large	15	2	0
Oranges, raw, whole, without peel and seeds, 1 orange	60	tr	0

FRUIT

FOOD/PORTION SIZE	CAL	FAT (g)	CHOL (mg)
Papayas, raw, 1/2-in. cubes, 1 cup	65	tr	0
Peaches, canned, heavy syrup, 1/2 peach	60	tr	0
Peaches, canned, juice pack, 1/2 peach	35	tr	0
Peaches, dried, uncooked, 1 cup	380	1	0
Peaches, frozen, sliced, sweetened, 1 cup	235	tr	0
Peaches, raw, whole, 2 1/2-in. diameter, 1 peach	35	tr	0
Peaches, Sliced, Lite, Libby's, 1/2 cup	50	0	na
Pears, Bartlett raw, with skin, 1 pear	100	1	0
Pears, Bosc raw, with skin, 1 pear	85	1	0
Pears, canned, heavy syrup, 1/2 pear	60	tr	0
Pears, canned, juice pack, 1/2 pear	40	tr	0
Pears, D'Anjou raw, with skin, 1 pear	120	1	0
Pears, Halves, Lite, Libby's, 1/2 cup	60	0	na
Pineapple, canned, heavy syrup, crushed/chunks, 1 cup	200	tr	0
Pineapple, canned, heavy syrup, slices, 1 slice	45	tr	0
Pineapple, canned, juice pack, crushed/chunks, 1 cup	150	tr	0
Pineapple, canned, juice pack, slices, 1 slice	35	tr	0
Pineapple, raw, diced, 1 cup	75	1	0
Plantains, without peel, cooked/boiled, sliced, 1 cup	180	tr	0
Plantains, without peel, raw, 1 plantain	220	1	0
Plums, canned, purple, heavy syrup, 3 plums	120	tr	0

FOOD/PORTION SIZE	CAL	FAT (g)	CHOL (mg)
Plums, canned, purple, juice pack, 3 plums	55	tr	0
Plums, raw, 1½-in. diameter, 1 plum	15	tr	0
Plums, raw, 2⅛-in. diameter, 1 plum	35	tr	0
Prunes, dried, cooked, unsweetened, 1 cup	225	tr	0
Prunes, dried, uncooked, 4 extra large or 5 large	115	tr	0
Raisins, seedless, ½-oz. packet, 1 packet	40	tr	0
Raisins, seedless, 1 cup	435	1	0
Raspberries, frozen, sweetened, 1 cup	255	tr	0
Raspberries, frozen, sweetened, 10 oz.	295	tr	0
Raspberries, in Lite Syrup, Birds Eye Quick Thaw Pouch, 5 oz.	100	1	0
Raspberries, raw, 1 cup	60	1	0
Rhubarb, cooked, added sugar, 1 cup	280	tr	0
Strawberries, frozen, sweetened, sliced, 1 cup	245	tr	0
Strawberries, frozen, sweetened, sliced, 10 oz.	275	tr	0
Strawberries, Halved, in Syrup, Birds Eye Quick Thaw Pouch, 5 oz.	90	0	0
Strawberries, raw, capped, whole, 1 cup	45	1	0
Strawberries, Whole, Lite Syrup, Birds Eye, 4 oz.	80	0	0
Tangerines, canned, light syrup, 1 cup	155	tr	0
Tangerines, raw, 2⅜-in. diameter, 1 tangerine	35	tr	0
Watermelon, raw, 4×8-in. wedge, 1 piece	155	2	0
Watermelon, raw, diced, 1 cup	50	1	0

Gelatins, Puddings, & Pie Fillings

FOOD/PORTION SIZE	CAL	FAT (g)	CHOL (mg)
All flavors, Gelatin, Jell-O, 1/2 cup (average)	80	0	0
All flavors, Gelatin, Low Calorie, D-Zerta, 1/2 cup (average)	8	0	0
All flavors, Gelatin, Sugar Free, Jell-O, 1/2 cup (average)	8	0	0
Banana Cream, Pudding & Pie Filling, Instant, Jell-O, with whole milk, 1/2 cup	160	4	15
Banana Cream, Pudding & Pie Filling, Jell-O, with whole milk, 1/6 pie (excluding crust)	100	3	10
Banana, Pudding & Pie Filling, Instant, Sugar Free Jell-O, with 2% milk, 1/2 cup	90	2	10
Butter Pecan, Pudding & Pie Filling, Instant, Jell-O, with whole milk, 1/2 cup	170	5	15
Butterscotch, Pudding & Pie Filling, Instant, Jell-O, with whole milk, 1/2 cup	160	4	15
Butterscotch, Pudding & Pie Filling, Instant, Sugar Free, Jell-O, with 2% milk, 1/2 cup	90	2	10
Butterscotch, Pudding & Pie Filling, Jell-O, with whole milk, 1/2 cup	170	4	15
Butterscotch, Pudding, Reduced Calorie, D-Zerta, with skim milk, 1/2 cup	70	0	0
Chocolate Fudge, Pudding & Pie Filling, Instant, Jell-O, with whole milk, 1/2 cup	180	5	15

FOOD/PORTION SIZE	CAL	FAT (g)	CHOL (mg)
Chocolate Fudge, Pudding & Pie Filling, Instant, Sugar Free, Jell-O, with 2% milk, 1/2 cup	100	3	10
Chocolate Fudge, Pudding & Pie Filling, Jell-O, with whole milk, 1/2 cup	160	4	15
Chocolate Fudge, Rich & Luscious Mousse, Jell-O, with whole milk, 1/2 cup	150	6	10
Chocolate, pudding, canned, 5-oz. can	205	11	1
Chocolate, pudding, instant, dry mix made with whole milk, 1/2 cup	155	4	14
Chocolate, Pudding & Pie Filling, Instant, Jell-O, with whole milk, 1/2 cup	180	4	15
Chocolate, Pudding & Pie Filling, Instant, Sugar Free, Jell-O, with 2% milk, 1/2 cup	100	3	10
Chocolate, Pudding & Pie Filling, Jell-O, with whole milk, 1/2 cup	160	4	15
Chocolate, Pudding & Pie Filling, Sugar Free, Jell-O, with 2% milk, 1/2 cup	90	3	10
Chocolate, Pudding, Reduced Calorie, D-Zerta, with skim milk, 1/2 cup	60	0	0
Chocolate, pudding, regular (cooked), dry mix made with whole milk, 1/2 cup	150	4	15
Chocolate, Rich & Luscious Mousse, Jell-O, with whole milk, 1/2 cup	150	6	10
Chocolate Tapioca Pudding, Jell-O Americana, with whole milk, 1/2 cup	170	5	15

GELATINS, PUDDINGS, & PIE FILLINGS

FOOD/PORTION SIZE	CAL	FAT (g)	CHOL (mg)
Coconut Cream, Instant Pudding & Pie Filling, Jell-O, with whole milk, 1/2 cup	180	6	15
Coconut Cream, Pudding & Pie Filling, Jell-O, with whole milk, 1/6 pie (excluding crust)	110	4	10
Custard, baked, 1 cup	305	5	278
Custard, Golden Egg, Mix, Jell-O Americana, with whole milk, 1/2 cup	160	5	80
Fruit Punch, Gelatin, Royal, 1/2 cup	80	0	0
Gelatin dessert, prepared with water, 1/2 cup	70	0	0
Gelatin, dry, 1 envelope	25	tr	0
Lemon, Gelatin, Royal, 1/2 cup	80	0	0
Lemon, Pudding & Pie Filling, Instant, Jell-O, with whole milk, 1/2 cup	170	4	15
Lemon, Pudding & Pie Filling, Jell-O, with whole milk, 1/6 pie (excluding crust)	170	2	90
Lime, Gelatin, Royal, 1/2 cup	80	0	0
Milk Chocolate, Pudding & Pie Filling, Instant, Jell-O, with whole milk, 1/2 cup	180	5	15
Milk Chocolate, Pudding & Pie Filling, Jell-O, whole milk, 1/2 cup	160	4	15
Orange, Gelatin, Royal, 1/2 cup	80	0	0
Pineapple Cream, Pudding & Pie Filling, Instant, Jell-O, with whole milk, 1/2 cup	160	4	15
Pistachio, Pudding & Pie Filling, Instant, Jell-O, with whole milk, 1/2 cup	170	5	15
Pistachio, Pudding & Pie Filling, Instant, Sugar Free, Jell-O, with 2% milk, 1/2 cup	100	3	10

FOOD/PORTION SIZE	CAL	FAT (g)	CHOL (mg)
Raspberry, Gelatin, Royal, 1/2 cup	80	0	0
Rice Pudding, Jell-O Americana, with whole milk, 1/2 cup	170	4	15
Rice, pudding, prepared with whole milk, 1/2 cup	155	4	15
Strawberry/Banana, Gelatin, Royal, 1/2 cup	80	0	0
Strawberry, Gelatin, Royal, 1/2 cup	80	0	0
Strawberry/Orange, Gelatin, Royal, 1/2 cup	80	0	0
Tapioca, pudding, canned, 5-oz. can	160	5	tr
Tapioca, pudding, prepared with whole milk, 1/2 cup	145	4	15
Vanilla, French, Pudding & Pie Filling, Instant, Jell-O, with whole milk, 1/2 cup	160	4	15
Vanilla, French, Pudding & Pie Filling, Jell-O, with whole milk, 1/2 cup	170	4	15
Vanilla, pudding, canned, 5-oz. can	220	10	1
Vanilla, pudding, instant dry mix made with whole milk, 1/2 cup	150	4	15
Vanilla, Pudding & Pie Filling, Instant, Jell-O, with whole milk, 1/2 cup	170	4	15
Vanilla, Pudding & Pie Filling, Instant, Sugar Free, Jell-O, with 2% milk, 1/2 cup	90	2	10
Vanilla, Pudding & Pie Filling, Jell-O, with whole milk, 1/2 cup	160	4	15
Vanilla, Pudding & Pie Filling, Sugar Free, Jell-O, with 2% milk, 1/2 cup	80	2	10

FOOD/PORTION SIZE	CAL	FAT (g)	CHOL (mg)
Vanilla, Pudding, Reduced Calorie, D-Zerta, with skim milk, 1/2 cup	70	0	0
Vanilla, pudding, regular (cooked) dry mix, made with whole milk, 1/2 cup	145	4	15
Vanilla, Tapioca, Pudding, Jell-O Americana, with whole milk, 1/2 cup	160	4	15

Gravies & Sauces

FOOD/PORTION SIZE	CAL	FAT (g)	CHOL (mg)
GRAVIES			
Beef, canned, 1 cup	125	5	7
Brown, from dry mix, 1 cup	80	2	2
Chicken, canned, 1 cup	190	14	5
Chicken, from dry mix, 1 cup	85	2	3
Mushroom, canned, 1 cup	120	6	0
SAUCES			
Barbeque sauce, see BAKING PRODUCTS AND CONDIMENTS			
Cheese, from dry mix, prepared with milk, 1 cup	305	17	53
Hollandaise, prepared with water, 1 cup	240	20	52
Soy sauce, see BAKING PRODUCTS AND CONDIMENTS			

FOOD/PORTION SIZE	CAL	FAT (g)	CHOL (mg)
Spaghetti, Extra Chunky, Mushroom and Green Pepper, Prego, 4 oz.	110	6	na
Spaghetti, Extra Chunky, Tomato and Onion, Prego, 4 oz.	140	6	na
Spaghetti, Plain, Prego, 4 oz.	140	6	na
Spaghetti, Ragu, 4 oz.	80	3	0
Spaghetti, Thick & Hearty, Ragu, 4 oz.	140	5	0
Spaghetti, with Meat, Homestyle, Ragu, 4 oz.	70	2	2
Spaghetti, with Meat, Prego, 4 oz.	150	6	na
Spaghetti, with Meat, Ragu, 4 oz.	80	3	0
Spaghetti, with Mushrooms, Prego, 4 oz.	140	5	na
Spaghetti, with Mushrooms, Ragu, 4 oz.	80	4	0
Spaghetti, with Mushrooms, Thick & Hearty, Ragu, 4 oz.	140	5	2
White, medium, from home recipe, 1 cup	395	30	32

Legumes

FOOD/PORTION SIZE	CAL	FAT (g)	CHOL (mg)
BEANS			
Black, dry cooked, drained, 1 cup	225	1	0
Chickpeas, cooked, drained, 1 cup	270	4	0
Great Northern, dry, cooked, drained, 1 cup	210	1	0
Lentils, dry, cooked, 1 cup	215	1	0

LEGUMES

FOOD/PORTION SIZE	CAL	FAT (g)	CHOL (mg)
Lima, dry, cooked, drained, 1 cup	260	1	0
Lima, Giant, Seasoned with Pork, Luck's, 7 oz.	230	7	na
Lima, immature seeds, frozen, cooked, drained: thick-seeded types (Ford-hooks), 1 cup	170	1	0
Lima, immature seeds, frozen cooked, drained: thin-seeded types (baby limas) 1 cup	190	1	0
Lima, Small Green, Seasoned with Pork, Luck's, 7.5 oz.	220	7	na
Mixed (Pinto & Great Northerns), Seasoned with Pork, Luck's, 7.25 oz.	200	5	na
Navies, Ole Fashion, Ranch Style, 7.5 oz.	160	2	na
Navy, Seasoned with Pork, Luck's, 7.5 oz.	230	7	na
October, Seasoned with Pork, Luck's, 7.5 oz.	220	7	na
Pea, (Navy), dry, cooked, drained, 1 cup	225	1	0
Pinto, dry, cooked, drained, 1 cup	225	1	0
Pinto, Premium, Ranch Style, 7.5 oz.	160	1	na
Pinto, Seasoned with Pork, Luck's, 7.5 oz.	220	6	na
Pinto, with Onions, Seasoned with Pork, Luck's, 7.5 oz.	220	6	na
Red kidney, canned, 1 cup	265	1	0
Red Kidney, Dark, Ranch Style, 7.5 oz.	170	1	na
Red Kidney, Seasoned with Pork, Luck's, 7.5 oz.	220	6	na
Red Kidney, Special Cook, Luck's, 7.5 oz.	190	4	na
Refried, canned, 1 cup	295	3	0
Snap, canned, drained, solids (cut), 1 cup	25	tr	0

FOOD/PORTION SIZE	CAL	FAT (g)	CHOL (mg)
Snap, cooked, drained, from frozen (cut), 1 cup	25	tr	0
Snap, cooked, drained, from raw (cut and French style), 1 cup	45	tr	0
Speckled Butter, Seasoned with Pork, Luck's, 7.5 oz.	230	8	na
Sprouts, (mung) raw, 1 cup	30	tr	0
Tahini, 1 tbsp.	90	8	0
White, with pork and sweet sauce, canned, 1 cup	385	12	10
White, with pork and tomato sauce, canned, 1 cup	310	7	10
White, with sliced frankfurters, canned, 1 cup	365	18	30

NUTS

FOOD/PORTION SIZE	CAL	FAT (g)	CHOL (mg)
Almonds, Blanched/Slivered/Whole/Sliced, Planters, 1 oz.	170	15	0
Almonds, Dry Roasted, Planters, 1 oz.	170	15	0
Almonds, Honey Roasted, Planters, 1 oz.	170	13	0
Almonds, shelled, slivered, packed, 1 cup	795	70	0
Almonds, shelled, whole, 1 cup	165	15	0
Brazil, shelled, 1 oz.	185	19	0
Cashew Halves, Oil Roasted, Planters, 1 oz.	170	14	0
Cashew Halves, Oil Roasted, Unsalted, Planters, 1 oz.	170	14	0
Cashew, salted, dry roasted, 1 cup	785	63	0
Cashew, salted, roasted in oil, 1 cup	750	63	0
Cashews, Dry Roasted, Planters, 1 oz.	160	13	0

LEGUMES

FOOD/PORTION SIZE	CAL	FAT (g)	CHOL (mg)
Cashews, Dry Roasted, Unsalted, Planters, 1 oz.	160	13	0
Cashews, Fancy, Oil Roasted, Planters, 1 oz.	170	14	0
Cashews, Honey Roasted, Planters, 1 oz.	170	12	0
Cashews & Peanuts, Honey Roasted, Planters, 1 oz.	170	12	0
Chestnuts, European, roasted, shelled, 1 cup	350	3	0
Coconut, dried, sweetened, shredded, 1 cup	470	33	0
Coconut, raw, $2 \times 2 \times 1/2$-in. piece	160	15	0
Coconut, raw, shredded or grated, 1 cup	285	27	0
Filberts (hazelnuts), chopped, 1 cup	725	72	0
Macadamia, roasted in oil, salted, 1 cup	960	103	0
Mixed, Deluxe, Oil Roasted, Planters, 1 oz.	180	17	0
Mixed, Dry Roasted, Planters, 1 oz.	160	14	0
Mixed, Dry Roasted, Unsalted, Planters, 1 oz.	170	15	0
Mixed, Oil Roasted, Planters, 1 oz.	180	16	0
Mixed, Oil Roasted, Unsalted, Planters, 1 oz.	180	16	0
Mixed, with peanuts, salted, dry roasted, 1 oz.	170	15	0
Mixed, with peanuts, salted, roasted in oil, 1 oz.	175	16	0
Nut Topping, Planters, 1 oz.	180	16	0
Peanuts, Cocktail, Oil Roasted, Planters, 1 oz.	170	15	0
Peanuts, Cocktail, Oil Roasted, Unsalted, Planters, 1 oz.	170	15	0

FOOD/PORTION SIZE	CAL	FAT (g)	CHOL (mg)
Peanuts, Dry Roasted, Planters, 1 oz.	160	14	0
Peanuts, Dry Roasted, Unsalted, Planters, 1 oz.	170	15	0
Peanuts, Honey Roasted, Dry Roasted, Planters, 1 oz.	160	13	0
Peanuts, Honey Roasted, Planters, 1 oz.	170	13	0
Peanuts, Oil Roasted, Salted, Planters, 1 oz.	170	15	0
Peanuts, Redskin, Oil Roasted, Planters, 1 oz.	167	15	0
Peanuts, roasted in oil, salted, 1 cup	840	71	0
Peanuts, Roasted-in-shell, Salted, Planters, 1 oz.	160	14	0
Peanuts, Roasted-in-shell, Unsalted, Planters, 1 oz.	160	14	0
Peanuts, Spanish, Dry Roasted, Planters, 1 oz.	160	14	0
Peanuts, Spanish, Oil Roasted, Planters, 1 oz.	170	15	0
Peanuts, Spanish, Raw, Planters, 1 oz.	150	12	0
Peanuts, Sweet 'N Crunchy, Planters, 1 oz.	140	8	0
Pecans, Chips/Halves/Pieces, Planters, 1 oz.	190	20	0
Pecans, halves, 1 cup	720	73	0
Pine, (pinyons), shelled, 1 oz.	160	17	0
Pistachio, dried, shelled, 1 oz.	165	14	0
Pistachios, Dry Roasted, Planters, 1 oz.	170	15	0
Pistachios, Natural, Planters, 1 oz.	170	5	0
Pistachios, Red, Planters, 1 oz.	170	15	0
Sesame Nut Mix, Dry Roasted, Planters, 1 oz.	160	12	0
Tavern, Planters, 1 oz.	170	15	0
Walnuts, black, chopped, 1 cup	760	71	0

LEGUMES

FOOD/PORTION SIZE	CAL	FAT (g)	CHOL (mg)
Walnuts, Black, Planters, 1 oz.	180	17	0
Walnuts, English or Persian, pieces/chips, 1 cup	770	74	0
Walnuts, English, Whole/Halves/Pieces, Planters, 1 oz.	190	20	0

PEAS

Black-eyed, dry, cooked, 1 cup	190	1	0
Split, dry, cooked, 1 cup	230	1	0

SEEDS

Pumpkin/squash kernels, dry, hulled, 1 oz.	155	13	0
Sesame, dry, hulled, 1 tbsp.	45	4	0
Sunflower, dry, hulled, 1 oz.	160	14	0
Sunflower Nuts, Dry Roasted, Planters, 1 oz.	160	14	0
Sunflower Nuts, Dry Roasted, Unsalted, Planters, 1 oz.	170	15	0
Sunflower Nuts, Oil Roasted, Planters, 1 oz.	170	15	0
Sunflower Seeds, Planters, 1 oz.	160	14	0

SOY PRODUCTS

Miso, 1 cup	470	13	0
Soybeans, dry, cooked, drained, 1 cup	235	10	0
Tofu, $2^1/_2 \times 2^3/_4 \times 1$-in. piece	85	5	0

Meat

FOOD/PORTION SIZE	CAL	FAT (g)	CHOL (mg)
BEEF			
Braised/simmered/pot roasted, bottom round, lean and fat, 3 oz.	220	13	81
Braised/simmered/pot roasted, bottom round, lean only, 2.8 oz.	75	8	75
Braised/simmered/pot roasted, chuck blade, lean and fat, 3 oz.	325	26	87
Braised/simmered/pot roasted, chuck blade, lean only, 2.2 oz.	170	9	66
Canned, corned, 3 oz.	185	10	80
Dried, chipped, 2.5 oz.	145	4	46
Ground, broiled, patty, lean, 3 oz.	230	16	74
Ground, broiled, patty, regular, 3 oz.	245	18	76
Heart, lean, braised, 3 oz.	150	5	164
Liver, fried, $6^{1}/_2 \times 2^{3}/_8 \times {}^{3}/_8$–in. slice, 3 oz.	185	7	410
Roast, oven cooked, eye of round, lean and fat, 3 oz.	205	12	62
Roast, oven cooked, eye of round, lean only, 2.6 oz.	135	5	52
Roast, oven cooked, rib, lean and fat, 3 oz.	315	26	72
Roast, oven cooked, rib, lean only, 2.2 oz.	150	9	49
Steak, sirloin, broiled, lean and fat, 3 oz.	240	15	77
Steak, sirloin, broiled, lean only, 2.5 oz.	185	10	64

MEAT

FOOD/PORTION SIZE	CAL	FAT (g)	CHOL (mg)
FRANKS & SAUSAGES			
Frankfurter, chicken, 1 frank	115	9	45
Franks, Beef, Oscar Mayer, 1 link	150	14	30
Franks, Eckrich, 1 frank	190	17	na
Franks, Jumbo Beef, Eckrich, 1 frank	190	17	na
Sausage, pork, brown/serve, browned, 1 link	50	5	9
Sausage, pork, frankfurters, cooked, 1 frank	145	13	23
Sausage, Pork, Jimmy Dean, 33g	140	13	na
Sausage, pork, links, 1 1-oz. pork link	50	4	11
Weiners, Oscar Mayer, 1 link	140	13	30
LAMB			
Chops, arm, braised, lean and fat, 2.2 oz.	220	15	77
Chops, arm, braised, lean only, 1.7 oz.	135	7	59
Leg, roasted, lean and fat, 3 oz.	205	13	78
Leg, roasted, lean only, 2.6 oz.	140	6	65
Loin, broiled, lean and fat, 2.8 oz.	235	16	78
Loin, broiled, lean only, 2.3 oz.	140	6	60
Rib, roasted, lean and fat, 3 oz.	315	26	77
Rib, roasted, lean only, 2 oz.	130	7	50
LUNCHEON MEATS			
Chicken, roll, light, 2 slices (1 slice = 1 oz.)	90	4	28
Bologna, Beef, Oscar Mayer, 28g	90	8	15
Bologna, Oscar Mayer, 15g	50	4	na
Bologna sausage, 2 1-oz. slices	180	16	31
Braunschweiger sausage, 2 1-oz. slices	205	18	89
Ham, chopped, 8-slice (6-oz.) pack, 2 slices	95	7	21

FOOD/PORTION SIZE	CAL	FAT (g)	CHOL (mg)
Ham, cooked, extra lean, 8-slice (8-oz.) pack, 2 slices	75	3	27
Ham, cooked, regular, 8-slice (8-oz.) pack, 2 slices	105	6	32
Pork, canned lunch meat, spiced/unspiced, 2 3×2×1/2-in. slices	140	13	26
Salami sausage, cooked, 2 1-oz. slices	145	11	37
Salami sausage, dry, 12-slice (4-oz.) pack, 2 slices	85	7	16
Sandwich spread, pork/beef, 1 tbsp.	35	3	6
Turkey, ham cured thigh meat, 2 slices (1 oz. each)	75	3	32
Turkey Bologna, Louis Rich Turkey Coldcuts, 28g	60	5	na
Turkey, ham cured thigh meat, 2 slices (1 oz. each)	75	3	32
Turkey Ham, Louis Rich Turkey Coldcuts, 21g	25	1	na
Turkey Ham, Smoked, Louis Rich Turkey Coldcuts, 28g	35	2	na
Turkey, loaf, breast meat, 8-slice (6-oz.) pack, 2 slices	45	1	17
Turkey, Oscar Mayer, 21g	21	1	10
Turkey Pastrami, Louis Rich Turkey Coldcuts, 23g	25	1	na
Vienna sausage, 7 per 4-oz. can, 1 sausage	45	4	8

PORK

Bacon, cured, cooked, Canadian, 2 slices	85	4	27
Bacon, cured, cooked, regular, 3 medium slices	110	9	16
Ham, Boiled, Oscar Mayer, 21g	25	1	15
Ham, canned, roasted, 3 oz.	140	7	35

MEAT

FOOD/PORTION SIZE	CAL	FAT (g)	CHOL (mg)
Ham (leg), fresh, roasted, lean and fat, 3 oz.	250	18	79
Ham (leg), fresh, roasted, lean only, 2.5 oz.	160	8	68
Ham, light cure, roasted, lean and fat, 3 oz.	205	14	53
Ham, light cure, roasted, lean only, 2.4 oz.	105	4	37
Loin chop, fresh, broiled, lean and fat, 3.1 oz.	275	19	84
Loin chop, fresh, broiled, lean only, 2.5 oz.	165	8	71
Loin chop, fresh, pan fried, lean and fat, 3.1 oz.	335	27	92
Loin chop, fresh, pan fried, lean only, 2.4 oz.	180	11	72
Rib, fresh, roasted, lean and fat, 3 oz.	270	20	69
Rib, fresh, roasted, lean only, 2.5 oz.	175	10	56
Shoulder cut, fresh, braised, lean and fat, 3 oz.	295	22	93
Shoulder cut, fresh, braised, lean only, 2.4 oz.	165	8	76

VEAL

FOOD/PORTION SIZE	CAL	FAT (g)	CHOL (mg)
Medium fat, cutlet, braised/broiled, 3 oz.	185	9	109
Medium fat, rib, roasted, 3 oz.	230	14	109

Mixed Dishes

FOOD/PORTION SIZE	CAL	FAT (g)	CHOL (mg)
ABC's & 1, 2, 3's with Mini Meatballs, Chef Boy-ar-dee, 7.5 oz.	240	9	na
Beefaroni, Chef Boy-ar-dee, 7.5 oz.	220	8	na
Chicken a la king, cooked, home recipe, 1 cup	470	34	221
Chicken and noodles, cooked, home recipe, 1 cup	365	18	103
Chicken Stew, Chef Boy-ar-dee, EZO, 7.5 oz.	140	5	na
Chicken, Sweet & Sour, La Choy, 3/4 cup	120	2	na
Chili con carne with beans, canned, 1 cup	340	16	28
Chop suey with beef and pork, home recipe, 1 cup	300	17	68
Chow Mein, Beef, La Choy, 3/4 cup	70	1	na
Chow mein, chicken, canned, 1 cup	95	tr	9
Chow mein, chicken, home recipe, 1 cup	255	10	75
Chow Mein, Chicken, La Choy, 3/4 cup	80	3	na
Chow Mein with Beef, Chun King Stir-Fry Entrees, 6 oz.	290	19	50
Chow Mein with Chicken, Chun King Stir-Fry Entrees, 6 oz.	220	11	45
Egg Foo Young, Chun King Stir-Fry Entrees, 5 oz.	140	8	140
Egg Noodle and Cheese Dinner, Kraft, 3/4 cup	340	17	50
Egg Noodle with Chicken Dinner, Kraft, 3/4 cup	240	9	35

MIXED DISHES

FOOD/PORTION SIZE	CAL	FAT (g)	CHOL (mg)
Hamburger Helper, Beef Noodle, without meat, 1/5 pkg.	140	2	na
Hamburger Helper, Cheeseburger Macaroni, without meat, 1/5 pkg.	180	5	na
Hamburger Helper, Lasagna, without meat, 1/5 pkg.	160	1	na
Lasagna Dinner, Chef Boy-ar-dee, 5.97 oz.	280	8	na
Macaroni and Cheese Deluxe Dinner, Kraft, 3/4 cup	260	8	20
Macaroni and Cheese Dinner, Kraft, 3/4 cup	290	13	5
Macaroni and Cheese Dinner, Spiral, Kraft, 3/4 cup	330	17	10
Macaroni and Cheese Family Size Dinner, Kraft, 3/4 cup	290	13	5
Macaroni & Cheese, Golden Grain, Quaker Oats, dry mix, 1.81 oz.	190	2	na
Macaroni & Cheese, Golden Grain, Quaker Oats, prepared, 1.81 oz.	190	2.1	3.7
Macaroni (enriched) and cheese, canned, 1 cup	230	10	24
Macaroni (enriched) and cheese, home recipe, 1 cup	430	22	44
Quiche Lorraine, 1 slice (1/8 8-in. diameter quiche)	600	48	285
Potpie, beef, home recipe, baked, 1 piece (1/3 9-in. pie)	515	30	42
Potpie, chicken, home recipe, baked, 1 piece (1/3 9-in. pie)	545	31	56
Ravioli, Hearty Beef, Franco-American, 7 1/2 oz.	290	11	na
RavioliO's, Beef, Franco-American, 7 1/2 oz.	250	7	na
Shells and Cheese Dinner, Velveeta, 3/4 cup	260	10	25

FOOD/PORTION SIZE	CAL	FAT (g)	CHOL (mg)
Spaghetti, American Style Dinner, Kraft, 1 cup	310	8	0
Spaghetti Dinner, Tangy Italian Style, Kraft, 1 cup	310	8	5
Spaghetti in tomato sauce with cheese, canned, 1 cup	190	2	3
Spaghetti in tomato sauce with cheese, home recipe, 1 cup	260	9	8
SpaghettiO's, Franco-American, 7½ oz.	170	2	na
Spaghetti with meatballs and tomato sauce, canned, 1 cup	260	10	23
Spaghetti with meatballs and tomato sauce, home recipe, 1 cup	330	12	89
Spaghetti with Meatballs, Franco-American, 7⅜ oz.	220	8	na
Spaghetti with Meat Sauce Dinner, Kraft, 1 cup	360	14	15
Spaghetti with Tomato Sauce, Franco-American, 7⅜ oz.	190	2	na
Stew, beef/vegetable, home recipe, 1 cup	220	11	71

Pasta

FOOD/PORTION SIZE	CAL	FAT (g)	CHOL (mg)
Macaroni and cheese dishes, *see* MIXED DISHES			
Macaroni, enriched, cooked, firm, hot, 1 cup	190	1	0
Macaroni, enriched, cooked, tender, cold	115	tr	0

PASTA

FOOD/PORTION SIZE	CAL	FAT (g)	CHOL (mg)
Macaroni, enriched, cooked, tender, hot	155	1	0
Noodle Roni Chicken Mushroom, Quaker Oats, dry mix, 1.20 oz.	130	2	na
Noodle Roni Chicken Mushroom, Quaker Oats, prepared, 1.20 oz.	134	2.4	19.4
Noodle Roni Fettucini, Quaker Oats, dry mix, 1.50 oz.	180	5	na
Noodle Roni Fettucini, Quaker Oats, prepared, 1.50 oz.	181	5.1	26.8
Noodle Roni Garlic Butter, Quaker Oats, dry mix, 1.50 oz.	170	4	na
Noodle Roni Garlic Butter, Quaker Oats, prepared, 1.50 oz.	172	4.2	29.2
Noodle Roni Herb Butter, Quaker Oats, dry mix, 1 oz.	110	3	na
Noodle Roni Herb Butter, Quaker Oats, prepared, 1 oz.	114	2.7	19.0
Noodle Roni Parmesano, Quaker Oats, dry mix, 1.20 oz.	140	3	na
Noodle Roni Parmesano, Quaker Oats, prepared, 1.20 oz.	135	2.9	18.9
Noodle Roni Pesto, Quaker Oats, dry mix, 1.20 oz.	130	2	na
Noodle Roni Pesto, Quaker Oats, prepared, 1.20 oz.	131	2.1	na
Noodle Roni Romanoff, Quaker Oats, dry mix, 1.50 oz.	170	4	na
Noodle Roni Romanoff, Quaker Oats, prepared, 1.50 oz.	168	4.1	22.6
Noodle Roni Stroganoff, Quaker Oats, dry mix, 2 oz.	220	6	na
Noodle Roni Stroganoff, Quaker Oats, prepared, 2 oz.	225	6.4	42.3

FOOD/PORTION SIZE	CAL	FAT (g)	CHOL (mg)
Noodles, chow mein, canned, 1 cup	220	11	5
Noodles, egg, enriched, cooked, 1 cup	200	2	50
Spaghetti, enriched, cooked, tender, hot, 1 cup	155	1	0
Spaghetti with sauce/meat, see MIXED DISHES			
Vermicelli, Creamette, Extra Thin Spaghetti, dry, 2 oz.	210	1	0

Poultry

FOOD/PORTION SIZE	CAL	FAT (g)	CHOL (mg)
Chicken, canned, boneless, 5 oz.	235	11	88
Chicken, liver, cooked, 1 liver	30	1	126
Chicken, roasted, flesh only, breast, 3 oz.	140	3	73
Chicken, roasted, flesh only, drumstick, 1.6 oz.	75	2	41
Chicken, stewed, flesh only, light and dark meat, 1 cup	250	9	116
Coldcuts, chicken or turkey, see LUNCHEON MEATS in MEAT			
Duck, roasted, flesh only, 1/2 duck	445	25	197
Frankfurters, chicken or turkey, see FRANKFURTERS & SAUSAGES in MEAT			
Turkey, gravy and turkey, frozen, 5-oz. pkg.	95	4	26
Turkey, patties, breaded, batter fried, 1 patty	180	12	40

FOOD/PORTION SIZE	CAL	FAT (g)	CHOL (mg)
Turkey, roasted, boneless, frozen, seasoned, light and dark meat, chunked, 3 oz.	130	5	45
Turkey, roasted, flesh only, 1 light and 2 dark, 3 pieces	145	4	65
Turkey, roasted, flesh only, dark meat, 4 pieces	160	6	72
Turkey, roasted, flesh only, light and dark meat, 1 cup	240	7	106
Turkey, roasted, flesh only, light meat, 2 pieces	135	3	59

Rice

FOOD/PORTION SIZE	CAL	FAT (g)	CHOL (mg)
Beef Flavor, Rice-A-Roni, Quaker Oats, prepared, 1.33 oz.	135	0.9	0.8
Brown, cooked, hot, 1 cup	230	1	0
Brown & Wild, Mushroom Recipe, Uncle Ben's, 1/2 cup	130	1	na
Brown & Wild, Rice-A-Roni, Quaker Oats, prepared, 1.16 oz.	121	1.5	0.7
Chicken Flavor, Rice-A-Roni, Quaker Oats, prepared, 1.33 oz.	136	0.9	0.8
Chicken Mushroom, Rice-A-Roni, Quaker Oats, prepared, 1.25 oz.	129	1.2	0.9
Chicken Vegetable, Rice-A-Roni, Quaker Oats, prepared, 1.20 oz.	124	0.9	na
Drumstick, Minute Rice Mix, 1/2 cup	120	0	0

FOOD/PORTION SIZE	CAL	FAT (g)	CHOL (mg)
Drumstick, Minute Rice Mix, with butter, 1/2 cup	150	4	10
Extra-long grain, Riceland, 1/2 cup	85	0	na
French Style, Birds Eye International Rice Recipes, 3.3 oz.	110	0	0
Fried Chinese, Rice-A-Roni, Quaker Oats, prepared, 1.04 oz.	106	0.9	0.3
Fried Rice, Minute Rice Mix, 1/2 cup	120	0	0
Fried Rice, Minute Rice Mix, with oil, 1/2 cup	160	5	0
Herb Butter, Rice-A-Roni, Quaker Oats, prepared, 1.04 oz.	105	0.8	1.2
Instant, ready-to-serve, hot, 1 cup	180	0	0
Italian Style, Birds Eye International Rice Recipes, 3.3 oz.	120	1	0
Long Grain & Wild, Minute Rice Mix, 1/2 cup	120	0	0
Long Grain & Wild, Minute Rice Mix, with butter, 1/2 cup	150	4	10
Long Grain & Wild, Original Recipe, Uncle Ben's, 1/2 cup	100	0	na
Long Grain & Wild, Rice-A-Roni, Quaker Oats, prepared, 1 oz.	100	0.3	0.3
Minute Rice, without salt or butter, 2/3 cup	120	0	0
Natural Long Grain, Uncle Ben's, Converted, 2/3 cup	120	0	na
Rib Roast, Minute Rice Mix, 1/2 cup	120	0	0
Rib Roast, Minute Rice Mix, with butter, 1/2 cup	150	4	10
Risotto, Rice-A-Roni, Quaker Oats, prepared, 1.50 oz.	157	1.4	2.0

RICE

FOOD/PORTION SIZE	CAL	FAT (g)	CHOL (mg)
Savory Broccoli AuGratin, Rice-A-Roni, Quaker Oats, prepared, 1.12 oz.	129	3.4	4.0
Savory Cauliflower AuGratin, Rice-A-Roni, Quaker Oats, prepared, 1.20 oz.	141	3.6	4.7
Savory Chicken Florentine, Rice-A-Roni, Quaker Oats, prepared, 1.07 oz.	108	0.8	0.5
Savory Creamy Parmesan & Herb, Rice-A-Roni, Quaker Oats, prepared, 1.22 oz.	145	4.2	6.9
Savory Garden Pilaf, Rice-A-Roni, Quaker Oats, prepared, 1.12 oz.	113	0.8	1.1
Savory Rice Pilaf, Rice-A-Roni, Quaker Oats, prepared, 1.45 oz.	147	0.9	0.7
Savory Spring Vegetable & Cheese, Rice-A-Roni, Quaker Oats, prepared, 1.22 oz.	141	3.5	5.5
Spanish Style, Birds Eye International Rice Recipes, 3.3 oz.	110	0	0
Spanish Style, Rice-A-Roni, Quaker Oats, prepared, 1.07 oz.	107	0.6	0.5
Stroganoff, Rice-A-Roni, Quaker Oats, prepared, 1.35 oz.	150	3	4.9
White, enriched, cooked, hot, 1 cup	225	tr	0
White, enriched, raw, 1 cup	670	1	0
Yellow, Rice-A-Roni, Quaker Oats, prepared, 2 oz.	196	0.5	0.6

Salad Dressing

FOOD/PORTION SIZE	CAL	FAT (g)	CHOL (mg)
Bacon & Buttermilk, Kraft, 1 tbsp.	80	8	0
Bacon, Creamy, Reduced Calorie, Kraft, 1 tbsp.	30	2	0
Bacon & Tomato, Kraft, 1 tbsp.	70	7	0
Bleu Cheese, 1 tbsp.	75	8	3
Bleu Cheese and Herb, Good Seasons Mix, prepared with oil and vinegar, 1 tbsp.	80	9	0
Bleu Cheese, Chunky, Kraft, 1 tbsp.	70	6	0
Bleu Cheese, Chunky, Reduced Calorie, Kraft, 1 tbsp.	30	2	0
Bleu Cheese, Lite, Less Oil, Wishbone, 1 tbsp.	40	4	5
Bleu Cheese, Reduced Calorie, Roka Brand, 1 tbsp.	14	1	5
Bleu Cheese, Roka Brand, 1 tbsp.	60	6	10
Buttermilk & Chives, Creamy, Kraft, 1 tbsp.	80	8	5
Buttermilk, Creamy, Kraft, 1 tbsp.	80	8	5
Buttermilk, Creamy, Reduced Calorie, Kraft, 1 tbsp.	30	3	0
Buttermilk, Farm Style, Good Seasons Salad Dressing Mix, made with whole milk and mayonnaise, 1 tbsp.	60	6	0
Caesar, Weight Watchers, 1 tbsp.	4	0	na
Cheese Garlic, Good Seasons Mix, prepared with vinegar and oil, 1 tbsp.	80	9	0
Cheese Italian, Good Seasons Mix, prepared with vinegar and oil, 1 tbsp.	80	9	0
Coleslaw, Kraft, 1 tbsp.	70	6	10

SALAD DRESSING

FOOD/PORTION SIZE	CAL	FAT (g)	CHOL (mg)
Creamy, Reduced Calorie, Rancher's Choice, 1 tbsp.	30	3	5
Cucumber, Creamy, Kraft, 1 tbsp.	70	8	0
Cucumber, Creamy, Reduced Calorie, Kraft, 1 tbsp.	30	3	0
Creamy, Rancher's Choice, 1 tbsp.	80	8	5
French, Catalina Brand, 1 tbsp.	70	6	0
French, Kraft, 1 tbsp.	60	6	0
French, Lite, Less Oil, Wishbone, 1 tbsp.	18	1	na
French, low calorie, 1 tbsp.	25	2	0
French, No Oil, Pritikin, 1 tbsp.	10	0	na
French, Reduced Calorie, Kraft, 1 tbsp.	25	2	0
French, regular, 1 tbsp.	85	9	0
French, Weight Watchers, 1 tbsp.	10	0	na
Garlic and Herbs, Good Seasons Mix, made with oil and vinegar, 1 tbsp.	80	9	0
Garlic, Creamy, Kraft, 1 tbsp.	50	5	10
Golden Caesar, Kraft, 1 tbsp.	70	7	0
Herb, Classic, Good Seasons Mix, made with vinegar and oil, 1 tbsp.	80	9	0
Home prepared, cooked type, 1 tbsp.	25	2	9
Italian, Creamy, Lite, Less Oil, Wishbone, 1 tbsp.	25	2	10
Italian, Creamy, Reduced Calorie, Kraft, 1 tbsp.	25	2	0
Italian, Creamy, with Real Sour Cream, Kraft, 1 tbsp.	60	6	0
Italian, Good Seasons Mix, made with oil and vinegar, 1 tbsp.	80	9	0
Italian, Lite, Good Seasons Mix, made with oil and vinegar, 1 tbsp.	25	3	0

FOOD/PORTION SIZE	CAL	FAT (g)	CHOL (mg)
Italian, Lite, Zesty, Good Seasons Mix, made with oil and vinegar, 1 tbsp.	25	3	0
Italian, low calorie, 1 tbsp.	5	tr	0
Italian, Mild, Good Seasons Mix, made with oil and vinegar, 1 tbsp.	90	9	0
Italian, No Oil, Good Seasons Mix, prepared with vinegar and water, 1 tbsp.	6	0	0
Italian, No Oil, Pritikin, 1 tbsp.	6	0	na
Italian, Oil-Free, Kraft, 1 tbsp.	4	0	0
Italian, Presto, 1 tbsp.	70	7	0
Italian, Reduced Calorie, Kraft, 1 tbsp.	6	0	0
Italian, regular, 1 tbsp.	80	9	0
Italian, Weight Watchers, 1 tbsp.	6	0	na
Italian, Zesty, Good Seasons Mix, made with oil and vinegar, 1 tbsp.	80	9	0
Italian, Zesty, Kraft, 1 tbsp.	70	8	0
Lemon Herb, Good Seasons Mix, made with oil and vinegar, 1 tbsp.	80	9	0
Mayonnaise type, 1 tbsp.	60	5	4
Miracle Whip, 1 tbsp.	70	7	5
Miracle Whip Light, Reduced Calorie, 1 tbsp.	45	4	5
Oil & Vinegar, Kraft, 1 tbsp.	70	7	0
Onion & Chives, Creamy, Kraft, 1 tbsp.	70	7	0
Reduced Calorie, Catalina Brand, 1 tbsp.	16	0	0
Red Wine Vinegar and Oil, Kraft, 1 tbsp.	50	4	0
Russian, Reduced Calorie, Kraft, 1 tbsp.	30	1	0
Thousand Island & Bacon, Kraft, 1 tbsp.	60	6	0

SNACKS

FOOD/PORTION SIZE	CAL	FAT (g)	CHOL (mg)
Thousand Island, Kraft, 1 tbsp.	60	5	5
Thousand Island, Lite, Less Oil, Wishbone, 1 tbsp.	40	3	10
Thousand island, low calorie, 1 tbsp.	25	2	2
Thousand Island, Reduced Calorie, Kraft, 1 tbsp.	30	2	5
Thousand island, regular, 1 tbsp.	60	6	4
Tomato Vinaigrette, Weight Watchers, 1 tbsp.	8	0	na
Tomato, Zesty, No Oil, Pritikin, 1 tbsp.	18	0	na
Vinegar and oil, home prepared, 1 tbsp.	70	8	0

Snacks

FOOD/PORTION SIZE	CAL	FAT (g)	CHOL (mg)
BARS			
Breakfast, Peanut Butter Chocolate Chip, Carnation, 1 bar	200	11	na
Breakfast, Peanut Butter Crunch, Carnation, 1 bar	190	10	na
Dipps, Caramel Nut, Quaker Oats, 1.10 oz.	148	6.4	1.8
Dipps, Chocolate Chip, Quaker Oats, 1 oz.	139	6.3	1.4
Dipps, Chocolate Fudge, Quaker Oats, 1.10 oz.	160	7.9	na
Dipps, Peanut Butter & Chocolate Chip, Quaker Oats, 1.15 oz.	174	10	na

FOOD/PORTION SIZE	CAL	FAT (g)	CHOL (mg)
Dipps, Peanut Butter, Quaker *Oats, 1.15 oz.*	170	9.1	1.8
Slender, Chocolate, Carnation, *2 bars*	270	14	na
Slender, Chocolate Chip, *Carnation, 2 bars*	270	14	na
Slender, Vanilla, Carnation, *2 bars*	270	15	na

CORN CHIPS

Bugles, 1 oz.	150	8	na
Corn chips, 1-oz. package	155	9	0
Doritos, Cool Ranch, 1 oz.	140	7	0
Doritos, Nacho Cheese, 1 oz.	140	7	0
Doritos, Salsa Rio, 1 oz.	140	7	0
Doritos, Toasted Corn, 1 oz.	140	6	0
Fritos Corn Chips, 1 oz.	150	9	0
Fritos Corn Chips, Crisp n' Thin, *1 oz.*	160	10	0
Tostitos, Sharp Nacho Cheese, *1 oz.*	150	9	0
Tostitos, Traditional, 1 oz.	140	8	0

DIPS

Acapulco, Ortega, 1oz.	8	0	0
Avocado (guacamole), Kraft, *2 tbsp.*	50	4	0
Bacon & Horseradish, Kraft, *2 tbsp.*	60	5	0
Blue Cheese, Kraft Premium, *2 tbsp.*	45	4	10
Clam, Kraft, 2 tbsp.	60	4	10
Cucumber, Creamy, Kraft *Premium, 2 tbsp.*	50	4	10
French Onion, Kraft, 2 tbsp.	60	4	0
Garlic, Kraft, 2 tbsp.	60	4	0
Green Onion, Kraft, 2 tbsp.	60	4	0
Jalapeño Pepper, Kraft, 2 tbsp.	50	4	0

SNACKS

FOOD/PORTION SIZE	CAL	FAT (g)	CHOL (mg)
Nacho Cheese, Kraft Premium, 2 tbsp.	50	4	10
Onion, Creamy, Kraft Premium, 2 tbsp.	45	4	10

FRUIT SNACKS

FOOD/PORTION SIZE	CAL	FAT (g)	CHOL (mg)
Fruit Roll-Ups, Banana, 1/2 oz.	50	1	na
Fruit Roll-Ups, Cherry, 1/2 oz.	50	1	na
Fruit Roll-Ups, Grape, 1/2 oz.	50	1	na
Fruit Roll-Ups, Strawberry, 1/2 oz.	50	1	na
Fruit Roll-Ups, Watermelon, 1/2 oz.	60	1	na
Fruit Wrinkles, 1 pouch	100	2	na
Fun Fruits, all shapes, 9 oz.	100	1	na

GRANOLA

FOOD/PORTION SIZE	CAL	FAT (g)	CHOL (mg)
Chocolate Chip, Chewy Granola Bar, Quaker Oats, 1 oz.	128	4.7	0.3
Chocolate Graham & Marshmallow, Chewy Granola Bar, Quaker Oats, 1 oz.	126	4.4	0.3
Honey & Oats, Chewy Granola Bar, Quaker Oats, 1 oz.	125	4.4	0.3
Nut & Raisin, Chunky, Chewy Granola Bar, Quaker Oats, 1 oz.	131	5.8	0.2
Oats n' Honey, Granola Bar, Nature Valley, 1 bar	120	5	na
Peanut Butter, Chewy Granola Bar, Quaker Oats, 1 oz.	128	4.9	0.3
Peanut Butter Chocolate Chip, Chewy Granola Bar, Quaker Oats, 1 oz.	131	5.7	0.3
Raisin Cinnamon, Chewy Granola Bar, Quaker Oats, 1 oz.	128	5.0	0.3

FOOD/PORTION SIZE	CAL	FAT (g)	CHOL (mg)
POPCORN			
Air-popped, unsalted, 1 cup	30	tr	0
Microwave, Butter, Orville Redenbacher, 4 cups	110	6	na
Microwave, Natural, Orville Redenbacher, 4 cups	110	7	na
Microwave, Natural, Planters, 3 cups (popped)	140	9	0
Pan, Regular, Jiffy Pop, 4 cups (popped)	130	6	0
Planters, 3 cups (popped)	20	0	0
Popped in vegetable oil, salted, 1 cup	55	3	0
Sugar syrup coated, 1 cup	135	1	0
POTATO CHIPS			
Lays, 1 oz.	150	10	0
Lays, Bar-B-Que, 1 oz.	150	9	0
O'Grady's, 1 oz.	150	9	0
O'Grady's, Au Gratin, 1 oz.	150	8	0
O'Grady's, Hearty Seasoning, 1 oz.	140	8	0
Potato chips, 10 chips	105	7	0
Pringles, 1 oz.	170	13	na
Pringles Light, Bar-B-Que, 1 oz.	150	8	na
Pringles Light, Ranch, 1 oz.	150	8	na
Pringles, Sour Cream n' Onion, 1 oz.	170	12	na
Ruffles, 1 oz.	150	10	0
Ruffles, Cajun Spice, 1 oz.	150	10	0
Ruffles, Sour Cream & Onion, 1 oz.	150	9	na
PRETZELS			
Enriched flour, 2¼-in. sticks, 10 pretzels	10	tr	0
Enriched flour, twisted, dutch, 1 pretzel	65	1	0

FOOD/PORTION SIZE	CAL	FAT (g)	CHOL (mg)
Enriched flour, twisted, thin, 10 pretzels	240	2	0
Mister Salty, Sticks, Butter Flavor, 90 pretzels	110	1	na

RICE CAKES

FOOD/PORTION SIZE	CAL	FAT (g)	CHOL (mg)
Barley & Oats, Quaker Oats, 0.32 oz.	34	0.3	0
Buckwheat, Quaker Oats, 0.32 oz.	35	0.3	0
Corn, Quaker Oats, 0.32 oz.	35	0.3	0
Multi-Grain, Quaker Oats, 0.32 oz.	34	0.4	na
Multi-Grain, Salt-Free, Quaker Oats, 0.32 oz.	35	0.4	0
Plain, Quaker Oats, 0.32 oz.	35	0.3	0
Rye, Quaker Oats, 0.32 oz.	34	0.4	0
Sesame, Quaker Oats, 0.32 oz.	35	0.3	0
Sesame, Salt-Free, Quaker Oats, 0.32 oz.	35	0.3	0
Wheat, Quaker Oats, 0.32 oz.	34	0.3	0

Soup

FOOD/PORTION SIZE	CAL	FAT (g)	CHOL (mg)
Bean with bacon, canned, condensed, prepared with = volume of water, 1 cup	170	6	3
Beef broth bouillon consume, canned, condensed, prepared with = volume of water, 1 cup	15	1	tr
Beef noodle, canned, condensed, prepared with = volume of water, 1 cup	85	3	5

FOOD/PORTION SIZE	CAL	FAT (g)	CHOL (mg)
Bouillon, dehydrated, unprepared, 1 packet	15	1	1
Chicken, cream of, canned, condensed, prepared with = volume of milk, 1 cup	190	11	27
Chicken, cream of, canned, condensed, prepared with = volume of water, 1 cup	115	7	10
Chicken, Lemon, Lipton Lite Cup-A-Soup, 6 oz.	45	1	na
Chicken noodle, canned, condensed, prepared with = volume of water, 1 cup	75	2	7
Chicken noodle, dehydrated, prepared with water, 1 packet	40	1	2
Chicken rice, canned, condensed, prepared with = volume of water, 1 cup	60	2	7
Clam chowder, Manhattan, canned, condensed, prepared with = volume of water, 1 cup	80	2	2
Clam chowder, New England, canned, condensed, prepared with = volume of milk, 1 cup	165	7	22
Minestrone, canned, condensed, prepared with = volume of water, 1 cup	80	3	2
Mushroom, cream of, canned, condensed, prepared with = volume of milk, 1 cup	205	14	20
Mushroom, cream of, canned, condensed, prepared with = volume of water, 1 cup	130	9	2
Onion, dehydrated, prepared with water, 1 packet	20	tr	0

FOOD/PORTION SIZE	CAL	FAT (g)	CHOL (mg)
Pea, green, canned, condensed, prepared with = volume of water, 1 cup	165	3	0
Tomato, canned, condensed, prepared with = volume of milk, 1 cup	160	6	17
Tomato, canned, condensed, prepared with = volume of water, 1 cup	85	2	0
Tomato & Herb, Lipton Lite Cup-A-Soup, 6 oz.	70	1	na
Tomato vegetable, dehydrated, prepared with water, 1 packet	40	1	0
Vegetable beef, canned, condensed, prepared with = volume of water, 1 cup	80	2	5
Vegetable, Oriental, Lipton Lite Cup-A-Soup, 6 oz.	30	1	na
Vegetarian, canned, condensed, prepared with = volume of water, 1 cup	70	2	0

Vegetables

FOOD/PORTION SIZE	CAL	FAT (g)	CHOL (mg)
ALFALFA			
Seeds, sprouted, raw, 1 cup	10	tr	0
ARTICHOKES			
Globe or French, cooked drained, 1 artichoke	55	tr	0

FOOD/PORTION SIZE	CAL	FAT (g)	CHOL (mg)
Hearts, Birds Eye Deluxe Vegetables, 3 oz.	30	0	0
Jerusalem, red, sliced, 1 cup	115	tr	0

ASPARAGUS

Canned, spears, 4 spears	10	tr	0
Cuts, Birds Eye Regular Vegetables, 3.3 oz.	25	0	0
Cuts & tips, cooked, drained, from raw, 1 cup	45	1	0
Cuts & tips, from frozen, 1 cup	50	1	0
Spears, Birds Eye Regular Vegetables, 3.3 oz.	25	0	0
Spears, cooked, drained, from raw, 4 spears	15	tr	0
Spears from frozen, 4 spears	15	tr	0

BAMBOO SHOOTS

Canned, drained, 1 cup	25	1	0

BEANS

Baby Lima, Birds Eye Regular Vegetables, 3.3 oz.	130	0	0
Fordhook Lima, Birds Eye Regular Vegetables, 3.3 oz.	100	0	0
Green, Cut, Birds Eye Regular Vegetables, 3 oz.	25	0	0
Green, French Cut, Birds Eye Deluxe, 3 oz.	25	0	0
Green, Italian, Birds Eye Regular Vegetables, 3 oz.	30	0	0
Green, Whole, Birds Eye Deluxe Vegetables, 3 oz.	25	0	0

VEGETABLES

FOOD/PORTION SIZE	CAL	FAT (g)	CHOL (mg)
BEETS			
Canned, drained, solids, diced or sliced, 1 cup	55	tr	0
Cooked, drained, diced or sliced, 1 cup	55	tr	0
Cooked, drained, whole, 2 beets	30	tr	0
Greens, leaves and stems, cooked, drained, 1 cup	40	tr	0
BROCCOLI			
Baby Sprouts, Birds Eye Deluxe Vegetables, 3.3 oz.	30	0	0
Chopped, Birds Eye Regular Vegetables, 3.3 oz.	25	0	0
Cooked, drained, from frozen, 1 piece (4½-5 in. long)	10	tr	0
Cooked, drained, from frozen, chopped, 1 cup	50	tr	0
Cuts, Birds Eye Regular Vegetables, 3.3 oz.	25	0	0
Florets, Birds Eye Deluxe Vegetables, 3.3 oz.	25	0	0
Spears from raw, cooked, drained, 1 cup, (½-in. pieces)	45	tr	0
Raw, 1 spear	40	1	0
Spear, medium from raw, cooked, drained, 1 spear	50	1	0
Spears, Birds Eye Regular Vegetables, 3.3 oz.	25	0	0
BRUSSELS SPROUTS			
Birds Eye Regular Vegetables, 3.3 oz.	35	0	0
Cooked, drained, from frozen, 1 cup	65	1	0
Cooked, drained, from raw, 1 cup	60	1	0

FOOD/PORTION SIZE	CAL	FAT (g)	CHOL (mg)
CABBAGE			
Chinese pak-choi, cooked, drained, 1 cup	20	tr	0
Chinese pe-tsai, raw, 1-in. pieces, 1 cup	10	tr	0
Common varieties, coarsely shredded or sliced, 1 cup	15	tr	0
Common varieties, cooked, drained, 1 cup	30	tr	0
Red, raw, coarsely shredded or sliced, 1 cup	20	tr	0
Savoy, raw, coarsely shredded or sliced, 1 cup	20	tr	0
CARROTS			
Baby, Whole, Birds Eye Deluxe Vegetables, 3.3 oz.	40	0	0
Canned, sliced, drained, solids, 1 cup	35	tr	0
Cooked, sliced, drained, from frozen, 1 cup	55	tr	0
Cooked, sliced, drained, from raw, 1 cup	70	tr	0
Raw, without crowns or tips, scraped, grated, 1 cup	45	tr	0
Raw, without crowns or tips, scraped, 1 cup	30	tr	0
CAULIFLOWER			
Birds Eye Regular Vegetables, 3.3 oz.	25	0	0
Cooked, drained, from frozen (flowerets), 1 cup	35	tr	0
Cooked, drained, from raw (flowerets), 1 cup	30	tr	0

VEGETABLES

FOOD/PORTION SIZE	CAL	FAT (g)	CHOL (mg)
Raw (flowerets), 1 cup	25	tr	0

CELERY
Pascal type, raw, large outer stalk, 1 stalk	5	tr	0
Pascal type, raw, pieces, diced, 1 cup	20	tr	0

COLLARDS
Cooked, drained, from frozen (chopped), 1 cup	60	1	0
Cooked, drained, from raw (leaves without stems), 1 cup	25	tr	0

CORN
Big Ears, Cob, Birds Eye Regular Vegetables, 1 ear	160	1	0
Little Ears, Cob, Birds Eye Regular Vegetables, 2 ears	130	1	0
On the Cob, Birds Eye Regular Vegetables, 1 ear	120	1	0
Sweet, Birds Eye Regular Vegetables, 3.3 oz.	80	1	0
Sweet, canned, cream style, 1 cup	185	1	0
Sweet, cooked, drained, from frozen, 1 ear (3½ in.)	60	tr	0
Sweet, cooked, drained, from raw, 1 ear (5 × 1¾ in.)	85	1	0
Sweet, cooked, drained, kernels, 1 cup	135	tr	0
Sweet, vacuum packed, whole kernel, 1 cup	165	1	0
Tender, Sweet, Birds Eye Deluxe Vegetables, 3.3 oz.	80	1	0

FOOD/PORTION SIZE	CAL	FAT (g)	CHOL (mg)
CUCUMBER			
Peeled slices ⅛-in. thick, (large 2⅛-in. diameter, small 1¾-in. diameter), 6 large or 8 small	5	tr	0
EGGPLANT			
Cooked, steamed, 1 cup	25	tr	0
ENDIVE			
Curly (including escarole), raw, small pieces, 1 cup	10	tr	0
GREENS			
Dandelion, cooked, drained, 1 cup	5	1	0
Mustard, without stems and midribs, cooked, drained, 1 cup	20	tr	0
Turnip, cooked, drained from frozen (chopped), 1 cup	50	1	0
Turnip, cooked, drained from raw (leaves & stems), 1 cup	30	tr	0
KALE			
Cooked, drained from frozen, chopped, 1 cup	40	1	0
Cooked, drained, from raw, chopped, 1 cup	40	1	0
KHOLRABE			
Thickened bulb-like stem, cooked, drained, diced, 1 cup	50	tr	0

FOOD/PORTION SIZE	CAL	FAT (g)	CHOL (mg)
LETTUCE			
Looseleaf (bunching varieties including romain or cos), chopped or shredded, 1 cup	10	tr	0
Butterhead, as Boston types, raw, 1 head (5-in. diameter)	20	tr	0
Butterhead, as Boston types, raw, leaves, 1 outer or 2 inner leaves	tr	tr	0
Crisphead, as iceberg, raw, ¼ of head, 1 wedge	20	tr	0
Crisphead, as iceberg, raw, head (6-in. diameter), 1 head	70	1	0
Crisphead, as iceberg, raw, pieces, chopped, shredded, 1 cup	5	tr	0
MIXED VEGETABLES			
Baby Carrots, Peas, Pearl Onions, Birds Eye Deluxe Vegetables, 3.3 oz.	50	0	0
Bavarian Green Beans Spaetzle, Birds Eye International Recipe, 3.3 oz.	110	6	10
Broccoli, Baby Carrots, Water Chestnuts, Birds Eye Farm Fresh Mix, 3.2 oz.	35	0	0
Broccoli, Carrots, Pasta, Birds Eye Combination Vegetables, 3.3 oz.	90	4	0
Broccoli, Cauliflower, Carrot, Birds Eye Farm Fresh Mix, 3.2 oz.	25	0	0
Broccoli, Corn, Red Pepper, Birds Eye Farm Fresh Mix, 3.2 oz.	50	0	0
Broccoli, Green Beans, Pearl Onions, Red Peppers, Birds Eye Farm Fresh Mix, 3.2 oz.	25	0	0

FOOD/PORTION SIZE	CAL	FAT (g)	CHOL (mg)
Broccoli, Red Peppers, Bamboo Shoots, and Straw Mushrooms, Birds Eye Farm Fresh Mix, 3.2 oz.	25	0	0
Brussels Sprouts, Cauliflower, Carrots, Birds Eye Farm Fresh Mix, 3.2 oz.	30	0	0
Cauliflower, Baby Carrots, Snow Pea Pods, Birds Eye Farm Fresh Mix, 3.2 oz.	30	0	0
Chinese Style, Birds Eye International Recipe, 3.3 oz.	80	5	0
Chinese Style, Birds Eye Stir-Fry Vegetables, 3.3 oz.	35	0	0
Chow Mein Style, Birds Eye International Recipe, 3.3 oz.	90	4	0
Corn, Green Beans, Pasta, Birds Eye Combination Vegetables, 3.3 oz.	110	5	0
Green Beans, French, Toasted Almond, Birds Eye Combination Vegetables, 3 oz.	50	2	0
Green Peas, Pearl Onions, Birds Eye Combination Vegetables, 3.3 oz.	70	0	0
Italian Style, Birds Eye International Recipe, 3.3 oz.	110	7	0
Japanese Style, Birds Eye International Recipe, 3.3 oz.	100	6	0
Japanese Style, Birds Eye Stir-Fry Vegetables, 3.3 oz.	30	0	0
Mandarin Style, Birds Eye International Recipe, 3.3 oz.	90	4	0
Mixed Vegetables, Birds Eye Regular Vegetables, 3.3 oz.	60	0	0
New England Style Vegetables, Birds Eye International Style, 3.3 oz.	130	7	0

VEGETABLES

FOOD/PORTION SIZE	CAL	FAT (g)	CHOL (mg)
Pasta Primavera Style, Birds Eye International Recipe, 3.3 oz.	120	5	5
Rice, Green Peas, Mushrooms, Birds Eye Combination Vegetables, 2.3 oz.	110	0	0
San Francisco Style, Birds Eye International Style, 3.3 oz.	100	5	0
Vegetables, mixed, canned, drained, solids, 1 cup	75	tr	0
Vegetables, mixed, frozen, cooked, drained, 1 cup	105	tr	0

MIXED VEGETABLES WITH SAUCE

	CAL	FAT (g)	CHOL (mg)
Broccoli, Cauliflower, Carrot, Cheese Sauce, Birds Eye Cheese Sauce Combination Vegetables, 5 oz.	100	5	5
Broccoli, Cauliflower, Creamy Italian Cheese Sauce, Birds Eye Cheese Sauce Combination Vegetables, 4.5 oz.	90	6	15
Green Peas, Potatoes, Cream Sauce, Bird's Eye Combination Vegetables, 2.6 oz.	130	6	0
Mixed Vegetables with Onion Sauce, Birds Eye Combination Vegetables, 2.6 oz.	100	5	0
Peas, Pearl Onion, Cheese Sauce, Birds Eye Cheese Sauce Combination Vegetables, 5 oz.	140	5	0

MUSHROOMS

	CAL	FAT (g)	CHOL (mg)
Cooked, drained, 1 cup	40	1	0
Canned, drained, solids, 1 cup	35	tr	0
Raw, sliced or chopped, 1 cup	20	tr	0

FOOD/PORTION SIZE	CAL	FAT (g)	CHOL (mg)
OKRA			
Pods, 3 × ⅝ in., cooked, 8 pods	25	tr	0
ONIONS			
Cooked, (whole or sliced), drained, 1 cup	60	tr	0
Small, Whole, Birds Eye Regular Vegetables, 4 oz.	40	0	0
Raw, chopped, 1 cup	55	tr	0
Raw, sliced, 1 cup	40	tr	0
Rings, breaded par-fried, frozen, prepared, 2 rings	80	5	0
Spring, raw, bulb (⅜-in. diameter) and white portion of top, 6 onions	10	tr	0
PARSLEY			
Freeze-dried, 1 tbsp.	tr	tr	0
Raw, 10 sprigs	5	tr	0
PARSNIPS			
Cooked, (diced or 2-in. lengths), drained, 1 cup	125	tr	0
PEAS			
Black-eyed, immature seeds, cooked, drained, from frozen, 1 cup	225	1	0
Black-eyed, immature seeds, cooked, drained, from raw, 1 cup	180	1	0
Frozen, cooked, drained, 1 cup	125	tr	0
Green, Birds Eye Regular Vegetables, 3.3 oz.	80	0	0

VEGETABLES

FOOD/PORTION SIZE	CAL	FAT (g)	CHOL (mg)
Green, canned, drained, solids, 1 cup	115	1	0
Pods, edible, cooked, drained, 1 cup	65	tr	0
Tender Tiny, Birds Eye Deluxe Vegetables, 3.3 oz.	60	0	0

PEPPERS

Hot chili, raw, 1 pepper	20	tr	0
Sweet, (about 5 per lb., whole) stem and seeds removed, 1 pepper	20	tr	0
Sweet, (about 5 per lb., whole) stem and seeds removed, cooked, drained, 1 pepper	15	tr	0

PICKLES

Cucumber, dill, medium whole, 1 pickle (3¾-in. long, 1¼-in. diameter)	5	tr	0
Cucumber, fresh-pack slices, 2 slices (1½-in. diameter, ¼-in. thick)	10	tr	0
Cucumber, sweet gherkin, small, 1 pickle (whole, about 2½-in. long, ¾-in. diameter)	20	tr	0

POTATOES

Baked (about 2 per lb. raw), flesh only, 1 potato	145	tr	0
Baked (about 2 per lb. raw), with skin, 1 potato	220	tr	0
Boiled (about 3 per lb. raw), peeled after boiling, 1 potato	120	tr	0
Boiled (about 3 per lb. raw), peeled before boiling, 1 potato	115	tr	0

FOOD/PORTION SIZE	CAL	FAT (g)	CHOL (mg)
French fry strip (2- to 3½-in. long), fried in vegetable oil, 10 strips	160	8	0
French fried strip (2- to 3½-in. long), oven heated, 10 strips	110	4	0
Sweet, candied, 2½ × 2-in. piece, 1 piece	145	3	8
Sweet, canned, solid packed, mashed, 1 cup	260	1	0
Sweet, cooked (baked in skin), 1 potato	115	tr	0
Sweet, cooked (boiled without skin), 1 potato	160	tr	0
Sweet, vacuum pack, 1 piece, 2¾ × 1 in.	35	tr	0

POTATO PRODUCTS

FOOD/PORTION SIZE	CAL	FAT (g)	CHOL (mg)
Au gratin, prepared from dry mix, 1 cup	230	10	12
Au gratin, prepared from home recipe, 1 cup	325	19	26
Hashed brown, prepared from frozen, 1 cup	340	18	0
Mashed, prepared from home recipe, milk added, 1 cup	160	1	4
Mashed, prepared from home recipe, milk and margarine added, 1 cup	225	9	4
Potato salad, prepared with mayo, 1 cup	360	21	170
Prepared from dehydrated flakes (without milk), water, milk, butter, salt added, 1 cup	235	12	29
Scalloped, prepared from dry milk mix, 1 cup	230	11	27
Scalloped, prepared from home recipe, 1 cup	210	9	29

VEGETABLES

FOOD/PORTION SIZE	CAL	FAT (g)	CHOL (mg)
PUMPKIN			
Canned, 1 cup	85	1	0
Cooked, from raw, mashed, 1 cup	50	tr	0
RADISHES			
Raw, stem ends and rootlets cut off, 4 radishes	5	tr	0
SAUERKRAUT			
Canned, solids and liquid, 1 cup	45	tr	0
SPINACH			
Canned, drained solids, 1 cup	50	1	0
Chopped, Birds Eye Regular Vegetables, 3.3 oz.	20	0	0
Cooked, drained, from frozen, leaf, 1 cup	55	tr	0
Cooked, drained, from raw, 1 cup	40	tr	0
Raw, chopped, 1 cup	10	tr	0
Souffle, 1 cup	220	18	184
Whole Leaf, Birds Eye Regular Vegetables, 3.3 oz.	20	0	0
SQUASH			
Summer (all varieties), cooked, sliced, drained, 1 cup	35	1	0
Winter (all varieties), cooked, baked, cubed, 1 cup	80	1	0
Winter, cooked, Birds Eye Regular Vegetables, 4 oz.	45	0	0
TOMATOES			
Canned, solids and liquid, 1 cup	50	1	0
Juice, canned, 1 cup	40	tr	0

FOOD/PORTION SIZE	CAL	FAT (g)	CHOL (mg)
Paste, canned, 1 cup	220	2	0
Puree, canned, 1 cup	105	tr	0
Raw, 2⅗-in. diameter (3 per 12-oz. pkg.), 1 tomato	25	tr	0
Sauce, canned, 1 cup	75	tr	0

TURNIPS

Cooked, diced, 1 cup	30	tr	0

VEGETABLES WITH SAUCE

Broccoli with Cheese Sauce, Birds Eye Cheese Sauce Combination Vegetables, 5 oz.	120	6	5
Broccoli with Creamy Italian Cheese Sauce, Birds Eye Cheese Sauce Combination Vegetables, 4.5 oz.	90	6	15
Brussels Sprouts with Cheese Sauce, Birds Eye Cheese Sauce Combination Vegetables, 4.5 oz.	110	6	5
Cauliflower with Cheese Sauce, Birds Eye Cheese Sauce Combination Vegetables, 5 oz.	110	6	5
Green Peas with Cream Sauce, Birds Eye Combination Vegetables, 2.6 oz.	120	6	0
Onions, Small, with Cream Sauce, Birds Eye Combination Vegetables, 3 oz.	110	6	0
Spinach, Creamed, Birds Eye Combination Vegetables, 3 oz.	60	4	0

Yogurt

FOOD/PORTION SIZE	CAL	FAT (g)	CHOL (mg)
Banana, Dannon, 1 cup	240	3	na
Blueberry, Dannon, 1 cup	240	3	na
Blueberry, Dannon Fresh Flavors, 1 cup	200	4	0
Blueberry, Lite n' Lively, 5 oz.	150	1	10
Blueberry, Yoplait, 6 oz.	190	3	na
Cherry, Yoplait 150, 6 oz.	150	0	5
Fruit-flavors, added milk solids, made with lowfat milk, 8 oz.	230	2	10
Plain, added milk solids, made with lowfat milk, 8 oz.	145	4	14
Plain, added milk solids, made with nonfat milk, 8 oz.	125	tr	4
Plain, Dannon, 1 cup	140	4	na
Plain, without added milk solids, with whole milk, 8 oz.	140	7	29
Raspberry, Dannon Fresh Flavors, 1 cup	200	4	na
Red Raspberry, Lite n' Lively, 5 oz.	140	2	10
Strawberry-Banana, Yoplait, 6 oz.	190	3	na
Strawberry, Dannon Fresh Flavors, 1 cup	200	4	na
Strawberry, Lite n' Lively, 5 oz.	150	2	10
Strawberry, Yoplait 150, 6 oz.	150	0	5
Strawberry, Yoplait Light, 6 oz.	90	0	5
Vanilla, Dannon, 1 cup	200	3	na
Vanilla, Yoplait 150, 6 oz.	150	0	5